MATTERS OF LIFE AND DEATH

First published in Great Britain in 1970
by Darton, Longman & Todd Limited
85 Gloucester Road, London SW7
© 1970 Edward Shotter, Francis Camps, Cicely Saunders,
J. Dominian, C. Murray Parkes, R. Y. Calne, W. J. Dempster,
G. R. Dunstan

Printed in Great Britain by Unwin Brothers Ltd, The Gresham Press,
Old Woking, Surrey, England.

ISBN 0 232 51114 4

MATTERS OF LIFE AND DEATH

By

Francis Camps, Cicely Saunders, J. Dominian,
C. Murray Parkes, R. Y. Calne, W. J. Dempster,
G. R. Dunstan

Edited by
Edward Shotter

Darton, Longman & Todd
London

CONTENTS

INTRODUCTION

Medical ethics can no longer be picked up on a ward round alone.
But there is no formal teaching on the making of moral decisions in
British medical schools; and the recent Royal Commission on
Medical Education made no recommendation on the subject. Indeed,
there is no accepted body of teaching on which such instruction could
be based. This series seeks to fill a well-recognised gap in medical
education but is addressed to a wider readership amongst those who
are prepared to reflect upon issues raised in the practice of
medicine.

Hitherto, there has been in the medical profession a general
consensus on the majority of major moral questions. In Europe at
least, the Hippocratic tradition and the Christian tradition of moral
theology have tended to support each other. This may be no longer
true; and ethics is too important a subject to leave to chance consideration. There is a growing realisation in medical schools that
the traditional ethical attitudes need further thought in the face of
modern therapy. The prolongation of life in unconscious patients,
the choice of recipients for renal dialysis or transplantation,
developments in genetics and surgical advances all pose new and
pressing problems both for the medical profession and for society.
Traditional moral theology is often ill-fitted to deal with these new
and sophisticated issues. Theological premises are not usually
appealed to when medical men discuss moral decisions. Indeed,
medical progress over the past three hundred years might be said to
be partly due to the acceptance of the cartesian dualism which re-
leased medicine from ecclesiastic control. There is good historical
precedent for the physician to resent any trespassing by the priest
in the realm of healing. On the other hand too many doctors still
think that co-operation between doctors and clergy means 'faith
healing'. They prefer that parsons should restrict their interest to
the soul, leaving the body to the physician.

One of the first signs that there was new thinking on the part of
the Church in medico-moral questions, and particularly in the way
they should be approached, was the appearance of the report[1] of
a small group of specialists in various fields, including theologians,
on some of the ethical problems raised by new medical techniques
of resuscitation and for keeping people alive—or the 'Prolongation
of Dying' as the *Lancet* has put it.[2] However, in 1966, before popular interest in medical ethics had been aroused by spectacular
developments in surgery, *The Times* medical correspondent wrote,

quoting Rostand, that 'Science has made us gods before we are
worthy of being men'. That, he wrote, 'was nearly thirty years ago;
what was then more fear than fact has now become a crisis. Almost
immeasurable medical progress has posed the community with
problems that will need all the skill of lawyers, philosophers and
theologians if the dignity of human life is to be maintained. '
Two years later, in an editorial, the *New Scientist*[3] called for 'a
code of conduct'. The writer, discussing chemical and biological
warfare, argued that the 'successful pursuit of knowledge, so widely
accepted as man's highest and finest need, can be twisted to totally
evil purposes. '

The medical profession, of course, has its own strict code of
conduct, but too often medical ethics seems to be more concerned
with questions of professional practice and etiquette than with moral
decisions. The Hippocratic Oath is no longer taken by newly qualified doctors; it is part of medical history, but there is little or no
teaching on the modern codes of Nurenberg, Geneva and Helsinki.
The debate on Lord Raglan's Bill to legalise voluntary euthanasia
showed that the demand for this did not come from the medical
profession itself. The majority of doctors who spoke opposed the
proposals, but it was the Bishop of Durham who called for 'training
in moral decision making'[4] in medical education, and supported
the work of the London Medical Group in this field.

Most of the contributors to this volume have lectured to clinical
medical students in the London teaching hospitals, at the invitation
of the London Medical Group, a student group for the study of issues
raised through the practice of medicine which concern the theologian, the philosopher and the sociologist. One purpose of this particular volume is to demonstrate the necessity of inter-dis-
ciplinary discussion of medico-moral questions. The time has
passed when either the medical profession itself or the Church or
the Law could act in isolation in these matters. However, the mere
presence of members of different professions does not guarantee
*inter*disciplinary discussion; it may lead to totally encapsulated
discussion, a compartmentalisation of the available knowledge. What
is required is that the different disciplines should learn to listen
to each other and thence to evaluate and apply the available insights.
Uncritical acceptance by one profession of the statements of repre-
sentatives of another may be worse than useless. It was largely as
a result of the available medical opinion that the Anglican bishops
decided, at the 1908 Lambeth Conference, to continue their opposition
to artificial means of contraception. Conversely, the presence of
medical advisers on the Papal Birth Control Commission was not

sufficient to persuade the Roman Catholic Church to change its position on birth control. The medical profession is no longer directly influenced by the dogmatic teaching of the churches. The most coherent system of medical ethics is the Roman Catholic: but it would appear that it carries little weight beyond its most strict adherents, and its philosophical basis is now in question. This is not to say that the insights of the theologian are valueless. A body of knowledge such as the Christian tradition of moral theology cannot reasonably be ignored in any discussion of medical ethics, since, as Lord Devlin points out in *The Enforcement of Morals,*[5] the Christian tradition has become part of the culture and social fabric of our society. Neither can the moral theologian afford to ignore the results of modern research in scientific medicine. However, there is a language barrier, which is unlikely to be bridged unless interdisciplinary studies become part of professional education. If medical education is a language course [6] then it is clear that its vocabulary needs to be extended by borrowing from other languages —as has been the case with all vital cultures. If public confidence in the practice of medicine is to be preserved, we must seek a new consensus on such questions as declaring a person to be dead, transplantation surgery, genetic engineering and clinical experimentation. It is the hope of the present editor that this small volume will contribute towards this process.

We have chosen the subject of death for a first volume, since it fulfils certain immediate needs. It may surprise the general reader to know that there tends to be something like a conspiracy of silence in the teaching hospitals about death. Doctors sometimes avoid discussing the topic almost as though it were a professional insult for a patient to die. Our choice also enables us to begin this series without yet another discussion of sex—which Jenkins [7] alleges is the only subject of which the Church is aware. Dr F. M. R. Walshe has remarked, 'no medical moral issue can ever get out of the pelvis'. This is no longer true, even if it were when written. Medical students have demonstrated that they are vitally interested in these questions and the following chapters are offered to a wider audience. They are published as 'work in progress': No attempt has been made to produce an artificial consensus. We hope that we have supplied sufficient footnotes to enable the non-medical reader to follow the thrust of the argument, although in Chapter 2 (Dr Cicely Saunders) we have given no further information on the drugs mentioned as this would have taken a great deal of space and still would not have added to the interest of the paper for the general reader. At the same time we hope that medical readers will excuse the statement of the obvious.

This book is a fruit of the lectures given since 1963 under the auspices of the London Medical Group, and it is intended as the first of a series. We must acknowledge with gratitude the enthusiasm of a growing number of medical teachers and students which has led to the development of this work. The present contributors have all given freely of their time and experience to develop the weekly lectures on medical ethics in the London Hospitals. Dr Martin Hayes-Allen, University College Hospital, and Dr Patrick Coyle, Charing Cross Hospital, both of whom as clinical medical students were officers of the London Medical Group, have made many helpful suggestions during the preparation of this volume. I am particularly grateful to Professor R. B. Welburn, Director of Surgery at the Royal Postgraduate Medical School for the advice he has given.

EFS

REFERENCES

1. *Decisions About Life & Death* Church Information Office, 1965.

2. *Lancet* 8 Dec. 1962 p. 1205.

3. *New Scientist,* 29th February 1968.

4. *Hansard.* Vol. 300 No. 50 23 March 1969.

5. O. U. P. 1968

6. R. Higgs, 'Learning to Communicate in Medicine' in *Progress in Medical Ethics* (London Medical Group) 1968.

7. Jenkins: *The Doctor's Profession,* S.C.M. Press 1949.

MATTERS OF LIFE AND DEATH

Francis Camps

In the past, death meant the end of life, but with modern advances in medical knowledge this is no longer the case. In this paper we shall be concerned with two aspects of death.

The first type of death is that which is inevitable—such as occurs with advanced carcinomatosis (Widespread cancer); or the complications, such as pulmonary infection, of a cerebro-vascular catastrophe ('Stroke') or 'uraemia' (Renal Failure) due to severe permanent renal damage. In such cases death is usually a slow process, sometimes with the death of particularly sensitive cells preceding somatic death or, occasionally, with some acute episode intervening, such as a pulmonary embolism (a blood clot blocking the blood vessels to the lungs). Usually, no attempt at resuscitation should be contemplated. Nevertheless, if such an ill-judged action were taken, it might be possible to maintain life, conscious or unconscious, with the use of sophisticated instruments, for a prolonged period.

The second type of death is that associated with abrupt, unexpected collapse. Perhaps the best recognised examples of this are those cases of cardiac arrest which occur during or shortly after surgical operations. Such instances lend themselves most easily to immediate resuscitation because all necessary facilities are available in the operating theatre. Another type, also amenable to resuscitation, is death due to electrocution, myocardial insufficiency (coronary artery disease) and cardiac arrest due to external stimuli (vagal inhibition). There is a further type, also associated with sudden collapse, in which there is an acute cardiovascular or cerebro-vascular catastrophe, such as a ruptured aneurysm of the abdominal aorta or cerebral haemorrhage. In these situations there is no real hope of recovery and, should resuscitation be successful, the patient is left in a permanently unconscious state or with some painful or psychologically impossible existence which would be covered by the quotation from Clough:

> 'Thou can'st not kill but should'st not strive
> officiously to keep alive.'

The subject of this discussion is 'death', but it is as well to appreciate that, in order to have death, there must be life: the problems associated with this are almost as complicated.

'God formed man of the dust of the ground and breathed into his nostrils the breath of life—and man became a living soul. '
                                                              Genesis 2 : 7

Life has been defined in many ways, none of which materially assists the problem about to be considered. For example,

'The property which differentiates a living animal or plant or a living portion of organic tissue from dead or non-living matter.'

immediately raises the question of somatic and cellular death, whilst

'Continuance of animate existence—opposite of death'

merely begs the question. Equally the definition of 'lifeless' as

'having no life; dead; insensible'

not only depends upon the definition of death but also does not even conform to it, unless it is accepted that all unconscious people are 'dead'—with which nobody can possibly agree. When one appreciates, in an age of rapid scientific and medical progress, the lack of precision in the use of words, together with legal definitions that are just as out of date, it looks very much as though the time to rethink and redefine has become overdue. As a relevant example: on a certain theological basis, life begins at the moment of conception, whilst on a legal definition a foetus is held to be viable after 28 weeks' gestation (Infant Life Preservation Act).

However, a foetus of under 28 weeks gestation which is on this definition 'non-viable' can be a live-birth 'having been completely expelled—showing signs of life or breathing'. In fact, so illogical is the definition of life (and still-birth) that a perfectly normal full-term child which is strangled whilst one foot is still in the vagina is legally a still-birth. A recent report of the British Medical Association has condemned this situation and has recommended that there should be a death certificate for 'still-birth'. Attention has been drawn to this in view of the problems of irreversible cerebral anoxia (the dead brain), to be discussed later, and a possible comparison with the absent brain of the anencephalic monster whose failure to survive, if due to an act of omission or commission, constitutes murder, by a literal interpretation of the law.

Examination of any textbook, old or new, will show that for the last hundred years at least a matter which has engaged the attention has been the time of death. Furthermore, in spite of a great deal of time and research, there has been a failure to produce a

solution to the problem. It may well be incapable of solution because there are too many unknown factors involved. A proper statistical appreciation would show this as another example of attempting
to resolve the problem by generalisation, particularly when the
original data are bedevilled by dogmatic statements handed down
from edition to edition on the time factors in relation to such
phenomena as fixation of hypostasis (R. v Emmett-Dunne) and appearance, persistence and loss of rigor mortis (R. v. Wallis).

Perhaps this state of affairs is in part due to the splendid isolation (or segregation) of the forensic pathologist from contact with
clinical and experimental medicine and similar subjects. The time
of death has also, on occasions, been confused with the time of attack
—victims may not die for hours or even days after a traumatic
incident.

It may be that these criticisms represent a 'defeatist' attitude
but there is worse to come, because the problems mentioned were
studied in the days when the practitioner believed that it was possible
to *establish* that death had occurred by:

> *vision* (the moving feather)
> *tactile sense* (the pulse)
> and *auditory perception* (the sounds in a stethoscope).

In view of the recognition of hypothermia (low body temperature),
as a modern alternative to narcolepsy (involuntary sleeping), and
certain dramatic incidences, such as recovery of consciousness in a
refrigerator or in a post-mortem room, it has become clear that
the traditional methods of proof of death must be reappraised. This
is not all: the power to resuscitate, ignored until recently, has been
used with moderate success, so that it is now impossible to say that
a person is dead even if the ECG (electrocardiograph—heart beat
tracing) and EEG (electroencephalograph—brain wave tracing) show
nothing, unless there is no intention to attempt resuscitation: a decision which might one day lead to action for negligence. But of
course with successful re-establishment of cardiac rhythm and
respiration, the possibility will still exist that the ultimate 'living'
result may prove to be merely a drain on the assets of the community. It is clear then that the definition 'live' (and here it is
obvious that consideration must be given to the unborn and new born
child) must be carefully linked with the definition of death.

It is, of course, those rare cases in which the individual is re-
suscitated yet not fully restored to life, but only to apparent normality, that receive widest publicity. There is little doubt that it is
the speed with which resuscitative measures are instituted that

dictates the result and this, in its turn, should be the responsibility of the person who has to weigh the pros and cons of even making or discontinuing the attempt. Let no mystery be made of the situation. It is possible with modern methods to maintain life—if by this is meant a beating heart and breathing lungs—for an almost indefinite time so that there is a body which will perform basic functions without being conscious. So, too, in the early period after the heart has been started, it is impossible to say what may happen. Even when at the time of 'death' the ECG and EEG waves were absent, after the heart has started, they will return.

The position, therefore, is easily understood. On the basis of one original definition which ran 'shows signs of life or breathes', 'death' has occurred and 'life' has been restored. However, there remains a 'body' which does not perform purposeful actions or speak or *apparently* recognise its surroundings. This state of affairs has been called 'a vegetable state'. It would be easy if the situation rested there, or even could be anticipated three months' hence, but this is not so. What is not yet known, although it may be a matter of 'guesswork', is whether the central nervous system is still functioning. In other words: how much can an unconscious person feel?

This question has a historical significance and was the basis of a controversial correspondence which arose at the time of the introduction of a humane method of decapitation by 'Dr. Guillotine'. It began in the 'Moniteur' on 20th May 1783, with an open letter by Sommering and Oesler as to how much the head felt after severance by the 'widow'. This, no doubt, stimulated Alexandre Dumas' romantic account of the execution of Marat's murderess, Charlotte Corday.

She was alleged to have blushed on both cheeks when her face was slapped by the executioner's assistant, Legros. In the heated discussion which followed, several cases were cited proving that there were reactions as well as several interesting explanations to disprove them. There is insufficient space to go into the details but although André Soubiran thought that Dumas had a vivid imagination, he commented: 'But all the same...' An example of the unreliability of eye-witnesses in moments of emotion is well shown in the three independent descriptions of the execution of Mary, Queen of Scots. All three eye-witnesses differ, except in one matter—that she was decapitated by a single blow. Objective evidence has shown that, on this point, they were all wrong.

Reverting to 'reception' during unconsciousness, there is evidence that in hypoglycaemic coma (Unconsciousness due to low concentration of sugar in the blood, for instance after an overdosage of Insulin in diabetes) the patient can appreciate what is happening without being able to speak and the same is said to occur in carbon monoxide poisoning. Thus, one cannot avoid asking whether it is an intact, functioning central nervous system which makes the difference between *true* life and death: in other words, *human life* means the presence of a 'mind'. It is impossible to define life by reference to one single factor for it involves both 'the body' and 'the mind'. Thus, it is impossible to deny that a person is alive if he still is, or is capable of being, mentally normal; and this applies even though he requires a respirator to maintain his respiration or a pacemaker to maintain his heartbeat. On the other hand, he might be said to be alive when, although possibly incapable of consciousness, he is still able to breathe without mechanical assistance. Here again we do not always know whether unconsciousness is synonymous with lack of appreciation. Under such circumstances, indeed, it would be murder to switch off the respirator in a case of poliomyelitis but a matter of doubt in a person whose brain might be so damaged that consciousness could never be regained. The latter conclusion, unless it is recognised, leads to the unrealistic position that a headless body would have to be kept from putrefaction by mechanical means, to the detriment of other conscious persons.

It must now be obvious that the importance of the time of death fades into the background in face of the problems produced by modern medicine. On a purely traditional basis, which must have been theological in origin, death was associated with departure of the soul from the body. The Oxford English Dictionary defines death as 'the final cessation of the vital functions' and the true significance of this definition lies in the word 'final', because now not only must the function *cease,* but it must also be incapable of being restored.

The present problems, still unappreciated by many, are in the main legal and ethical and will have to be resolved by the law. The present confused situation is due not only to modern methods of resuscitation but also to the re-examination of the old techniques, which followed upon 'the development of precise methods for evaluating pulmonary function[1]. Traditional methods of artificial respiration have been reassessed and, in some cases, replaced by what might be called 'modern' techniques, were it not for the fact that nothing is new. Reference to the Second Book of Kings will show:

> And he said unto his father—My head! My head! and he said unto the lad . . . . . carry him to his mother . . . . . he sat on her knees and then died.

He went and lay upon the child and put his mouth upon his mouth and his eyes upon his eyes and his hands upon his hands, and he stretched himself upon the child and the flesh of the child waxed warm.

Then he returned and walked into the house to and fro and went up and stretched himself upon him—and the child sneezed seven times and the child opened its eyes.

II Kings, 4:19, 34 and 35.

This is a classical description of modern mouth-to-mouth resuscitation and it is no accidental coincidence for there is an earlier reference:

v. 21   'He stretched himself upon the child three times . . . . . '

v. 22   '. . . . . and the soul of the child came into him again and he revived. '

I Kings 17:21-22.

From this there can be no doubt that the word 'final' (in the OED definition of death) is highly relevant, and that it will apply even more to cardiac massage. Yet, to 'final' must also be added 'irreversible' as will be seen later. The following cases are illustrative:-

CASE I

'A man was admitted to hospital for gastrectomy. The operation was successfully completed and he was returned to the ward. A short time later he collapsed from cardiac arrest. External cardiac massage was immediately carried out, without result—direct massage by opening the chest was then done. As a result, the heart restarted and severe bleeding was noticed from the abdominal drainage tube. Quite properly, it was decided to operate again and it was then found that, as a result of the pressure used in cardiac massage, there was a severe rupture of the liver, which was repaired. In spite of this he died. At the Inquest, the Coroner asked the pathologist the cause of death and the reply was that it depended upon when he died. i.e. either when the cardiac arrest occurred or after the repair of the liver   The Coroner correctly decided the cause of death was the ruptured liver.'

CASE II

'Following the Christmas holiday, work on an artesian well was recommenced at the Zoological Gardens. On removing the covers in the 'pit', the workers, who had failed to take precautions entirely, collapsed and died of carbon dioxide poisoning. Two keepers in the Reptile House, who went to their rescue, also collapsed, and, whilst one died, the other survived, remaining unconscious for a year. He ultimately died of a respiratory infection and, at autopsy, was found to have complete degeneration of his central nervous system, including optic atrophy. It is still a matter of investigation as to whether this was due to irreversible anoxia or specifically carbon dioxide poisoning but since then two cases of recovery have shown retinal changes which appear to be permanent. '

From this it can be seen that, on the basis of the survival of the cardiovascular and respiratory systems, such cases are 'alive', but the central nervous system, at some stage, is 'dead'. If the 'mind' be part of the central nervous system, then death took place when the degenerative process was irreversible. If such a concept be accepted then then the following definition of 'death' can be postulated.

'The final cessation of the vital functions as shown by irreversible changes in the central nervous system.'

This does not, however, completely solve the problem of whether, having once decided that a person is 'legally' dead, it is permissible to destroy the cardiovascular and respiratory systems by, for example, stopping a mechanical respirator, which by any definition, would be 'homicide'. A more practical approach is made by Hogan, who suggests that unless some decision is taken on these lines, there may be so many respirators 'tied up' that those who might benefit would not be able to do so.

So far, the whole argument may have appeared too theoretical but the consequences are in fact more practical as can be seen in the following case:-

CASE III

'One Saturday evening at 11 pm, as a result of an assault, a man called Potter sustained a fractured base of the skull from falling

backwards and striking his head on the pavement. He was admitted
to hospital and a blood-clot from the surface of the brain was removed. His wife was told that he would be alright. At about 11 am
on the Sunday morning, his respiration ceased and an artificial respirator maintained his breathing. At 5 pm his wife was asked for
permission for a kidney to be removed to transplant into the body of
another man whose previous graft had failed. To this she agreed
under the impression that the kidney would be removed after death.
(No one has the right to give consent for any operation which will
benefit someone else, but only to benefit himself). At about 11 am on
Monday, the unconscious man, with his heart beating, his kidneys
functioning and his breathing mechanically maintained, was taken to
the operating theatre where his kidney was removed and transplanted
into another person. As soon as the removal was completed, the
respirator was immediately stopped and his body taken to the
mortuary.

At the subsequent inquest, a verdict of Manslaughter was returned against the doctor and he was committed to stand his trial.
The evidence given by the surgeon was that Potter was dead when the
respiration ceased (ie at 11 am on Sunday) and, by the pathologist,
from his findings at the autopsy, that death was inevitable. Legal
opinion was quite definite that whoever stopped the respirator could
be guilty of homicide. The case was, therefore, submitted to the
Magistrates who accepted that death was when the respirator was
stopped and dismissed the case on a submission of *Novus actus.'*

This case has been subsequently reviewed in the Medico-Legal
Journal in which Lord Brock, the eminent cardiac surgeon, is quoted
as follows:-

'..... at least the heart and respiration must cease and not be
capable of revival before life is extinct .....'

It is also said that there can be no distinction between medical and
legal death and the ultimate decision must lie with the doctor, which,
to quote an eminent judge referring to medical evidence 'might lead
to trial by doctors!

'Thou shall'st not kill, but needst not strive officiously to
keep alive' may still be in the mind of the clinician as his hand
moves towards the switch which controls the respirator. Conversely
patients may feel: 'Whilst there's life, there's hope'; and 'The
American Way of Death', quotes a Funeral Directors' Journal:
'embalming makes it quite certain you will not be buried alive'.

TO SUMMARISE:

The situations which may arise fall empirically into groups in which are involved the disciplines of *theology*—the spirit, the mind, the soul and the hereafter; of *medicine*—ethical behaviour, which is closely associated with obedience to the *law* accompanied by a scientific and humane approach. Clinical responsibility is related to the interests of the individual and the community. The interests of the law, which must be the ultimate arbiter, will lie in such matters as inheritance and in the framing of definitions that will fit in with a modern concept of life and death. The Law must control those decisions of the medical profession which may be induced by an ever-increasing scientific curiosity. All of us must become fully aware that we are now rapidly approaching a time when replacement of any organ may be possible. We must envisage a time when not only may a person have his heart and lungs replaced with those of somebody else but also his brain. If it may not be so long before it is possible to acquire a new mind, why not a psychopathic personality?

Although it may seem a masterpiece of understatement, it would appear that a new definition of death is not only a matter of importance but of some urgency. So, too, is the decision as to who shall decide when life has ceased to exist.

'But come he slow or come he fast,
It is but death that comes at last.'

REFERENCES

1.   Conroe—*Artificial Respiration.*

THE NATURE AND MANAGEMENT OF TERMINAL PAIN

Cicely Saunders

Chronic pain and, still less, terminal pain, are not just extensions in time of something that is qualitatively the same as acute pain. Terminal pain has no useful function, serving neither as a warning nor for protection, but, when it occurs, merely adding to a deteriorating illness something that is really an illness in itself, one that has to be considered and treated as such. Here we are faced with pain that is not just an event, or a series of events, such as the pain of injury or after operation, but rather a situation in which the patient is, as it were, held a captive. The hardest thing about it for him is that it appears to be meaningless as well as endless, often bringing with it a sense of isolation and despair.

Many patients who die of cancer have no pain or indeed little discomfort at all and some patients with other terminal illnesses have greater pain for a longer period. Yet the picture of misery that comes into our minds as well as into that of the public when we think of some deaths from cancer does have a foundation in fact. Riding, [1] who has been running a Pain Clinic for several years, writes: The 'wretchedness of the patient with cancer pain, even at a relatively early stage, is very greatly different from that seen in most other pain. Postherpetic neuralgia (pain following shingles) of many years' duration does not lead to the degeneration of personality, the indifference to personal appearance and the total preoccupation with the pain itself that cancer causes. It may be thought that this is obviously the case because the victim knows or suspects that he has cancer. This explanation is not adequate because when such pain is alleviated then, despite continuing loss of weight and weakness, the wretchedness and misery vanish'.

The typical pain of cancer, as he points out, and as we have observed ourselves, is a constant pain which may or may not have exacerbations. It frequently disturbs patients at night or may practically forbid sleep and, although it is usually helped for a time by mild analgesics (pain-killing drugs) and/or hypnotics (drugs to make one drowsy), if the disease progresses into the true intractable pain the story the patient gives is of less and less relief for shorter and shorter periods. When asked to describe such pain, patients tend to move into realms other than the merely physical and say such things as, 'Well, doctor, it began in my back but now it seems that all of me is wrong', and we hear such comments as, 'It seemed so strange, no-one seemed to want to look at me'. Or, 'Will you turn me out if I can't get better?'

These and other patients quoted from tape recordings used phrases typical of many. One elderly woman, on being asked about the pain before admission, replied simply, 'Pain? It was *all* pain;'— this means more than just the pain of skeletal metastases (deposits of cancer in bone), severe as it certainly was in her case: it means the pain of being alone and of realising that you can no longer cope and it means lost independence and curtailed activity, as well as anorexia (loss of appetite) sleeplessness and depression. Others speak, over and over again, of their need for 'attention' and their feelings of rejection. Such patients are extremely sensitive to any feelings we may entertain that 'there is nothing more to be done' and are aware if we withdraw, however subtly, from true contact with them. But many of those who are anxious *not* to withdraw still feel helpless and doubtful of their ability to relieve such pain. There can be great difficulty in discovering the path between too much and too little treatment, between the too speedy or the too late resource to powerful analgesics. This is a problem that has many facets. The whole picture is coloured by the problem of the patient's awareness of the nature of his illness, and the two different questions of his diagnosis and his prognosis and by the doctor's own views as well as by his family's anxiety. All the problems of emotional distress accompanying deteriorating illness are there whether the patient knows its true nature or not, but they are all accentuated by the anxiety that unresolved and unexpressed problems can impose. And, in their turn, they are all helped by a positive approach to the treatment of pain and to the many other symptoms that may accompany terminal illness. A positive attitude to these minor problems affects the approach to the major ones and talk about symptoms, which may be a way out of talking about more serious concerns, can also be a way in, or a way of conveying reassurance on a much deeper level. The communication without words, or at least with indirect ones, is often the most important communication that takes place. And such talk also gives the opportunity for recognising the moment when the real question is not, 'What do you tell your patients?' but rather 'What do you let your patients tell you?'

The aim of such communications and of such treatment is that the patient should both be relieved of his distress and remain himself, helped not only to die peacefully but also to *live* until he dies.

And, in doing so, find his 'own' death. The battle now is not for recovery but for relief coupled with dignity and enjoyment—that the
patient should neither be swamped by distress nor smothered by
treatment but remain alive as a person, leaving his family with those
good memories which do so much to help them through bereavement.

This treatment can be summed up under three headings: listening, attention to detail, and skill and confidence in handling analgesics
and other drugs.

LISTENING TO THE PATIENT

In the first place—listening. Listening in order to analyse the situation and to attend, as a person ready to be aware, not only of the
nature of the pain on the physical level but also of its implications
for this individual, with his own culture and background, past experience and present anxieties. A patient who said, 'It seemed as if the
pain went with me talking', speaks for very many. Another who
said, 'It seems that all of me is wrong', is speaking of an inter-
related complex of physical, emotional and social problems while
she also expresses her need for a feeling of security and meaning.
This 'total pain', the pain which demands the patient's 'total preoccupation', calls for understanding and an approach along each of
these lines. The patients who keep saying to us, 'I knew I needed
attention', do not only refer to the physical side of their problems
but to the rest also. Such complaint is not always really justified;
many of us tend to blame something or someone other than ourselves when we are unwilling to admit that the problem is that our
own body is letting us down or that, in one way or another, the fault
is in ourselves. But too often it really is true. One doctor refers
to his Pain Clinic as 'a refuge for the rejected' and another says,
'These patients are so often jettisoned by their doctors.' Both of
them emphasise that their main contribution may just be the fact
that they are able to listen. Such ability includes a readiness for
real concern as well as time available.

ATTENTION TO DETAIL

Secondly, attention to detail. Attention not only to the details of the
story and to all the facets of the physical part of the pain, but also
to the various symptoms that may accompany it and to their treatment. Sometimes patients will complain bitterly of a minor trouble

in order to distract the attention of the doctor (and their own) from more major concerns that are too threatening to look at. But so often it *is* the apparently smaller thing that is the biggest problem. So much 'pain' can be relieved by symptomatic treatment, by nursing measures, control of any intercurrent infections, (infection occurring during the course of another disease) attention to diet and so on. Those who offer lists of such remedies are often hesitant because of their very simplicity. Each will garner his own that work for him and we all need a combination of enquiry, imagination and persistence. There is hardly anything that we cannot try to improve and very often we will succeed. To come to a patient with several different ideas to help anorexia, nausea, dyspnoea (difficulty with breathing), insomnia, incipient incontinence—perhaps above all constipation—makes the visit very much easier for us as well as more profitable for the patient.

To say that there is 'nothing more to be done', as Smithers[2] has pointed out, is 'inexcusable and seldom, if ever, true'. Symptomatic treatment, so wrong when definitive treatment is possible, is here not only demanded, but also extremely rewarding.

HANDLING OF DRUGS

Thirdly, skill and confidence in handling analgesics and their adjuvants. The skill of knowing when to begin, what to choose, what route and what regime to use, what combination of drugs to employ. When to begin? Not all patients with terminal malignant disease have pain and there are few studies to give us any guide as to the number we should expect to give these problems. Turnbull,[3] asked a group of gynaecologists the incidence of intractable pain in patients with carcinoma of cervix and received answers varying from 'negligible' to '100%'. His own records of 100 patients seen consecutively during the same period and in the same area indicated 38% with intractable pain and 14 probable cases. Aitken Swan,[4] interviewing families after a patient's death from cancer found that, while in 18% of cases a qualified statement was made concerning pain and its relief, 20% of the relatives gave distressing descriptions of pain and lack of relief, corresponding to popular opinion. Another survey of patients at home carried out more recently by Wilkes[5] showed that half of his nearly 400 patients had no difficulty in relief but that 24 of the 32 who had difficulties lasting for longer than 3/12 had severe pain. As he says, 'You cannot calibrate suffering', and indeed, we cannot, neither in time span nor in its intensity for the individual;

one week may be an intolerably long time and one patient is a fully significant figure, both for that person and for those who care for him. Certainly among the many patients who have no pain, or even little discomfort, there are many who have severe pain over long periods of time.

We do not resort automatically to narcotics (drugs producing insensibility) the moment this diagnosis is made but equally certainly we should do something about the pain as soon as it becomes a matter of complaint. The patient should be accustomed to expect relief rather than to expect pain from the very beginning of his downhill course. The present impact of pain is greatly influenced both by past experience of it and the future expectation which is based on such experience. If fear is aroused it will immediately enhance severe pain and the tendency to rely upon drugs. Fear increases pain by tension and by emphasising its threat, while if severe pain is allowed to occur the dramatic relief that is associated with the injection that dispels it can easily lead to problems of dependence. Such crises should be anticipated and avoided whenever possible.

This early relief can be carried out with mild analgesics, given regularly if pain is already constant, and many have remarked how useful they remain, often right through the whole course of such an illness. A well tried remedy in which the patient has confidence may also remain a standby as a supplement to much stronger drugs at a later stage. In spite of the newer drugs that are continually becoming available, aspirin, paracetamol and codein, and their combinations, remain the standbys. The dangers of aspirin in this situation are not great and are certainly acceptable. Soluble preparations seem more satisfactory for many patients, particularly when dissolved in an antacid mixture, which in its turn may be mildly laxative, and the combination with codein seems undoubtedly to have a good deal to offer, especially for patients with pain from skeletal metastases. In this group, dextropropyphene (Doloxene) is extremely popular in the United States in spite of its unimpressive performance in clinical trials. Its elegant presentation and still more the confidence with which it is given by so many people illustrate the importance of factors other than pure drug action. The placebo effect (effect produced by a drug other than its known pharmacalogical effect) has been described as 'the most important single factor in the treatment of human suffering'. It is indeed of very great importance and not merely a factor to be allowed for in clinical trials. Enthusiasm, instruction and the doctor's own confidence often do more to relieve pain than any drugs, although for such pain as we are considering a combination of them all is usually needed. It is because enthusiastic interest is so often denied to the patient with terminal cancer that his pain may be so fraught with misery.

Treatment of pain may often overlap with definitive palliative treatment at this stage and this in turn will often lead to the relief of pain. Discussion of the various possibilities is outside the scope of this discussion but it is our experience and that of others that expectation of such relief to come should not prevent adequate use of analgesics temporarily. Patients rarely wish to continue with drugs once the pain goes. It is our experience in seeing many patients on admission for terminal care that they have more often had too little than too much in the way of analgesics. More frequently they have had too many of unsuitable sedatives.

The use of mild analgesics should usually be combined with symptomatic treatment and possibly with small doses of sedatives or tranquillisers. There are many to choose from. Most psychiatrists give chlorpromazine as their drug of choice in the phenothiazine group. In our experience it is the best drug for patients who are at all confused or restless (used most easily in syrup form), but it tends to be too heavily sedative for alert patients or at earlier stages of illness. The varying degrees of sedation that accompany the use of different drugs of this group may often depend upon the doses in which they are commonly presented but it is always worth while to try several in order to discover the one which suits the individual patient. It is not surprising that it should be more difficult to match the right tranquillizer and its dose to the needs of the individual than it is to choose the correct analgesics. In both cases the right choice should avoid too much sedation.

There is insufficient space here to mention most of the other possible drugs, but amytal remains the favourite barbiturate for most doctors and often rivals the phenothiazines in controlling anxiety and also the fear that accompanies dyspnoea. Chlordiazepoxide (librium) is often worth trial for patients with anxiety and tension, and depression in most of these patients responds much more readily to the relief of pain and to the drugs already mentioned than to the anti-depressants so far available.

Relief, like pain, is self-perpetuating. Early, imaginative and confident handling of all these adjuvants will add many to the number of patients who never need strong analgesics at all.

There are many drugs in the moderate range of analgesics which may appear to be equipotent in trials but which have very different effects and side effects among patients. Once again we have to find a middle way, the way between having too few drugs on our

list to help the rare patient who reacts adversely to our well tried
favourites or, on the other hand, a list so long that we do not have
sufficient experience with any drug to use it with proper confidence
and discrimination. The art of giving analgesics, mild or powerful,
lies in handling drugs whose effects and side effects we know, balanc-
ing the dose to the need of the individual patient and adding adjuvants
as they are called for and our own confidence and interest at all
times. There are many analgesics for moderately severe pain. We
found that the most useful were methadone, dipipanone, levorphanol
and phenazocine. All of these should be used orally whenever this is
possible. We also used nepenthe, to which soluble aspirin or codein
co. were added as the mixture was used, but found that we used less
and less of it as we developed the use of very small doses of other
narcotics. Some departments find it an extremely satisfactory mixture, especially for bone pain, but it by no means suits all patients.

All these drugs may be sufficient for the control of severe pain
but they are also useful for pain of moderate severity if given in
correct dosage. It is often valuable to use a small dose of a stronger
analgesic rather than a larger dose of a less powerful drug, for there
is likely to be less incidence of side effects. Each of these drugs
may cause anorexia and nausea with some patients and should often
be combined with an anti-emetic (drug which prevents vomitting).
Some are presented in mixed preparation but it is better to discover
the patient's own best combination of drugs.

On the whole one has less need in hospital to learn the use of
the drugs available as suppositories but there is obviously a place
for these in general practice. Oxycodone is sometimes found to be
a most useful analgesic by this route and chlorpromazine and pro-
chlorpermazine are also widely used in this way. The drugs of the
phenothiazine group are valuable adjuncts when dealing with pain of
moderate severity. Whether or not they should accurately be described as potentiators of analgesics they certainly act in combination with them to give patients greater comfort. Even if their effect
is merely sedative, this is helpful in relieving the emotional and
reactive component of the total pain complex. One of them, however—
methotrimeprazine (Veractil)—has been shown to be a strong analgesic itself. In our experience it is likely to be rather too sedative
if used as the only analgesic for severe pain, but it makes an excellent adjuvant to the opiates.

It has been suggested that elderly patients should be rather
heavily sedated by the drugs of this group and only given the stronger
analgesics 'when the pain breaks through'. Although elderly patients
are very prone to pain on movement they seem to be less suscep-

tible to the typical steady pain of cancer and for many these drugs are sufficient for relief and comfort. We must be very careful to be alert to the presence of pain when a patient is scarcely able to complain of it; I am sure that most of us have a recollection of how a toothache or other pain may intrude upon our dreams before it finally wakes us up. On the whole, patients very much dislike being made to feel 'dopey'. For severe pain nothing has yet really replaced the opiates but there continues to be a lack of adequate comparisons of the effects and side effects of the different members of this group of drugs and of the synthetic groups also. Long term studies are almost entirely lacking. Different regimes of drug giving and the effects of different routes have still to be compared and this work is greatly needed to give us the facts upon which we can base rational practice and teaching.

Here again, however, patients (and doctors) have their idiosyncracies. Some prefer omnopon to morphine, others find that diamorphine gives relief with fewer side effects than any other drug in this situation. We used it extensively at St. Joseph's Hospice, in doses ranging from 2.5 mgm. upwards and found that nothing else made our patients so free from pain while they still remained alert and serene. It should be tried for those patients who are made sleepy or nauseated by the other opiates and those whose mental distress is not helped by the synthetic drugs. It can be particularly valuable for women, who are more often nauseated than men by other opiates, and for those for whom morphine is dysphoric.

While we still wait and plan for definitive trials between these drugs in the situation in which they will be used, it is of the greatest importance that whatever strong analgesics are used should be rightly handled. It is the performance of the physician above all that avoids the onset of dependence. If drugs are well managed from the early stage of such illness we rarely need large doses of drugs. Narcotics are too often introduced too late, at too high a dose level or by injection when oral dosage would be sufficient—as well as far easier to arrange at home. Diamorphine was given in over 900 doses to 48 patients who remained with us for more than three months. Over two-thirds of these doses were given orally in the popular mixture with cocaine and gin according to a somewhat flexible 4 hourly routine. Only 9 patients ever needed more than a 10 mgm. dose and 19 had 5 mgm. or less throughout the time they had this mixture. Atmosphere, confidence and the ready use of adjuvants lead to such a pattern of dosage and no-one should be led to withhold needed drugs from another patient in a different situation just because of hearing of such figures. There are patients whose extending lesions give increased pain and tolerance *does* sometimes occur. It is rarely helpful to increase the dose beyond some 60 mgm. of morphine or its equivalent (and such a large dose should rarely be necessary) nor to reduce the interval between doses to less than 3 hours. At such a stage we should increase sedatives or tranquillizers, which in any case should have been introduced long before with such a patient. Anticipation and imagination should avoid the real crises of this nature and certainly should avoid the very heavy sedation that obliterates the patient's personality and can reduce him to a mere uncomplaining residue of himself.

The prospect that drugs will inevitably fail to control such pain at the end haunts relatives, often from the very first moment of knowing the patient's diagnosis and they—and often the patient as well—need a great deal of reassurance that this will not be allowed to happen. A patient who had an unexpected remission at a very late stage of her illness wrote afterwards that her worst suffering was in waiting for the pain that in fact never came. There is often some misunderstanding concerning the danger and the nature of dependence upon narcotics and other powerful analgesics in such illness. Many patients are denied the relief of these drugs or they are withheld until a late stage, after much suffering has already been endured, because of fear that it may happen. Those who work among these patients extensively find it rarely occurs. Physical dependence without underlying emotional disorder may be common but is in any case easily terminated and is not really a dependence problem. Psychical dependence, however, does matter, even if it lasts only for a few days and we must never say blandly that 'addiction is not a problem at this stage'. Emotional dependence and the endless longing for injections can make a patient's last days a nightmare that his family will find hard to forget—and it can be avoided. This very rarely occurs when drugs are given to a regular schedule but when it has happened or if a patient has been admitted in such a state we have found that the addition of amiphenazole is a help in management. In spite of the fact that many of the original claims made for this drug have not been substantiated by later workers, in our experience there is a place for its use as an adjuvant when such problems occur.

The regime in which all these powerful analgesics are given is of paramount importance. The typical pain of terminal cancer is constant in character, even when it has exacerbations. Constant pain calls for constant control and that means some form of regular giving of drugs. Here the usual teaching that doses of any such drug should be as widely spaced as possible does not apply. Drugs should now be given to prevent pain from occurring rather than to control it once it is present. Pain is the strongest antagonist to the drugs given to suppress it and it is of cardinal importance that neither its threat nor its presence should make a patient have to ask continually for relief. If he does this, he is reminded each time of his dependence upon the drugs and upon the person who gives them to him. If instead his analgesic is given regularly, with a slightly permissive or relaxed schedule, so that no-one is obsessively clock-watching, and is given in a dose carefully assessed to cover just a little longer than the chosen period, pain can be forgotten and the spiral of self-perpetuation, dependence and misery is never initiated. We have found over and over again that the same dose can be used effectively for weeks and months, and such experience is not unique. Of course, constant attention is always needed to be certain that the degree of pain has not altered and that the dose should be adjusted accordingly. Pain may increase as metastatic lesions spread but it frequently diminishes at the end and the dose may need reducing or the interval between doses lengthening, although this should never be done abruptly.

No discussion of the control of physical symptoms, or of the emotional distress of such pain, would be complete without mentioning the use of alcohol, one of the best sedatives for these patients and an excellent adjuvant in the relief of pain. Above all, it has the great advantage of the pleasure and gratification that accompany it, not to mention the possibilities for social exchange. A dose shared with the relatives, if not with the doctor, may be more efficacious as well as more convivial than any other medication. I remember telephoning the family doctor of a patient who had been able to return home from St. Joseph's and who had died some months later to ask if he had had to increase the dose of diamorphine in his mixture. 'No', said the doctor, 'but we pushed the whiskey up a fair bit.'

That the final comment on the control of terminal pain should be about the importance of social exchanges for these patients serves to underline one of the most important factors in their continued relief. Every kind of suffering is intensified by isolation, and terminal pain perhaps shows this with exceptional vividness. Neither drugs nor procedures nor anything else we may offer will ever take the place of interest and attention. And it must not be attention that is produced as a technique but one that expresses the real commitment of one person to another.

Some extracts follow from a conversation between the writer and a young woman with metastic carcinoma from a carcinoma of breast, under 6 weeks before her death. During the stay with us she had diamorphine for over 5 months by mouth, at 10 mgm. or less, approximately 4 hourly, all the time, and then had 10 mgm. by injection for her last 19 days. She is here describing her memories of her pain before admission and of its relief, and she also discussed her views on 'knowing' about her illness. I think that her alertness and the way she made a positive achievement of this part of her life came through in her tone of voice. That such achievements should be made is the aim and the reward of all our treatment of terminal pain.

Dr. S: How bad was the pain—that you—were feeling in such need?

Patient: I would say that the pain was so bad that I dreaded anyone touching me and when anyone knocked my bed or came near me the first thing I said to them—'Please don't touch me. Please don't move me'.

Dr. S: So that it was something that really got on top of you—it was really bad.

Patient: Oh yes. I—I—I would say that—it was an obsession in a way because it was all round me. I would lie still thinking: 'Well, I won't bring it on I will just lie still' and the mere fact of everything you did—if you coughed, if you sneezed, if you went to lift something or moved something, you would find it, you would have it.

Dr. S: How quickly did what I give you begin to work and help?

Patient: .... I think that within three days I would say I was very comfortable indeed. It seemed to be that there was something between me and the pain. It was like a nice thing wrapped round me. Because I never, never, felt it—I never felt the bones hurting me. I felt comfortable for the first time for a long, long time.

This was taken $4\frac{1}{2}$ months after admission; throughout that time the Diamorphine Mist. had remained at 10 mgs., although the adjuvants had been changed from time to time.

REFERENCES

1. Riding J. E. (1966) The outpatient pain clinic. *J. Roy Coll. Surg.* Ireland. 2. 279.

2. Smithers D. W. A Clinical Prospect of the Cancer Problem. E and S Livingstone (1960).

3. Turnbull, F. (1954) Intractable Pain. *Proc. Roy. Soc. Med.* 47, 155.

4. Aitken-Swan, J. (1959) Nursing the late cancer patient at home. The family's impressions. *Practitioner,* 183, 64.

5. Wilkes, E. (1965) Terminal cancer at home. *Lancet* i. 799.

FACING DEATH

J. Dominian

The theme of my paper has developed slowly. Some few years ago
I was treating an intelligent man, in his early thirties who was mor-
bidly preoccupied with death, his own pending disintegration. He
was an anxious person who suffered a great deal from these recurrent fears. At this stage of the proceedings I remembered
thinking about Christ and his attitude to death. I suppose the simi-
larity of age had something to do with this but I did not pursue it
any further.

This patient was not however an isolated example of patients
preoccupied with fears of death. Men and women of all ages, but
particularly in their teens, twenties and thirties come repeatedly
to my clinic complaining spontaneously of these feelings. Gradually
I began to ask specifically for such fears and little by little a clinical picture emerged. These men and women had certain features
in common. They were frequently of an anxious disposition. This
could well be ascribed to their constitutional make up and related
to genetic influences. With persistent uniformity they lacked a
clear sense of their personal identity. This is a technical term
and an explanation is indicated. By identity I mean a self awareness, a separate existence from parents which is sufficiently free
from anxiety and fear to allow the development of personal relationship without having to turn to parents or parent substitutes for
emotional support. A separate identity does not only need this
minimum emotional independence but also an equivalent acceptance
of self as a person worthy to receive and give love in an exchange
with others. A minimum awareness of an independent and lovable
self with a sense of direction and purpose are some of the vital
elements of a personal identity and these characteristics develop
in the bosom of a stable family where the child recognises itself
in the process of growth as a person, acknowledged, accepted and
wanted by the parents for its own sake. It is through the formation
of these early human bonds that the child discovers itself and
others and learns gradually to possess itself and freely give itself
to others. Unstable home situations deny the normal development
of an identity and the sciences of psychiatry and psychology have
been accumulating slowly the causes and patterns of these sources
of instability.

Coupled with this absence of a clear identity is a recurrent fear of personal disintegration of annihilation expressed in such terms of depersonalisation as: 'I fear that something terrible will happen' or 'nothing would be left of me'. Intimately associated with these feelings is the dread of the unknown, up or down there in pre Bishop of Woolwich language and the terror of leaving behind the objects and people who are sources of comfort and support.

This personality structure and feelings are a frequent clinical picture and as the numbers I saw increased I thought again about Christ. His approach to death was at the opposite pole of this continium. It could be said that He almost looked forward to it. He certainly spoke about it with equanimity and sombre anticipation.

Mark 8: 31 writes 'And he began to teach them that the Son of Man was destined to suffer grieviously, to be rejected by the elders and the chief priests and the scribes and to be put to death, and after three days to rise again and he said all this quite openly'.

In John 10. 14 we find 'I am the good shepherd, I know my own and my own know me, just as the Father knows me and I know the Father and I lay down my life for my sheep'.

In John 13:19 'I tell you this now, before it happens so that when it does happen you may believe that I am He'.

In Mark 9:31 'The Son of Man will be delivered into the hands of men; they will put him to death and three days after he has been put to death he will rise again'.

These and other passages exemplify Our Lord's calm anticipation of the central event in His life. There was no fear of the unknown. He knew He was going to the Father and there was no terror of leaving behind those with whom He was related.

By now a theme was developing in my mind. Such a clear cut view of death handled with such little disturbance presupposes, if my view is correct, a strong and definitive identity.

I am well aware of the danger of looking for what one wants in the Scripture to support a particular point of view. The texts provide an abundance of material which can be variously interpreted. There is, however, indisputable evidence indicating that Christ possessed an identity which showed the characteristics of certainty, security, self acceptance and an overwhelming capacity to love and be loved.

At a very early stage in the Gospel of St. Luke there is a remarkable passage. On the return from the feast of the Passover at the age of twelve his parents lost him. They returned to Jerusalem and found him in the temple. 'My child, why have you done this to us? See how worried your father and I have been, looking for you'.

'Why were you looking for me?', he replied, 'Did you not know that I must be busy with my Father's affairs?' But they did not understand what he meant. (1)

Long before his ministry started Christ indicates His close relationship to the Father and it is in this intimate union that he finds and expresses most clearly His own identity as a beloved Son with a specific mission. Here we are in the midst of the mystery of the Incarnation. We know little about Christ's relationship with Mary and Joseph. The references to the former are few. Such as they are they show respect, care and concern, especially at the crucifixion; but at times there is a powerful redirection of emphasis from his human situation to God the Father. The woman who raises her voice in the crowd to say 'Happy the womb that bore you and the breast you sucked' is not contradicted but the reply 'Still happier (are) those who hear the word of God and keep it' is an emphatic assertion of priorities in relationships. Again in Luke when his mother and his brothers came looking for him but could not reach him the reply to those who pointed out their presence was curt. 'My mother and my brothers are those who hear the word of God and put it into practice'.(2) Christ does not reject his mother and his love for her is indicated in the Crucifixion narrative of St. John in which he takes care to leave her in the care of his beloved disciple. This brief episode says all that we need to know of how much he cared for her. But there is no escaping the fact that his only significant relationship was with his Father. With God the Father there is a constant dialogue in which Christ received indisputable affirmation of his identity, and the measure of love that his Father entertains for him. At his baptism there is an early affirmation. 'And a voice spoke from heaven, This is my beloved son with whom I am well pleased'. (3) Thus at the beginning of his messianic mission there is an unequivocal declaration of the intimate relationship between Father and Son and the total approval by the former of the work of the latter. Christ affirms that he draws his life from the Father. 'As I, who am sent by the living Father, myself draw life from the Father, so whoever eats me will draw life from me'. (4)

The closeness between himself and the Father is to be seen in a number of passages particularly in the gospel of St. John. When the Pharisees questioned his integrity he showed no trepidation in his reply.

'You judge by human standards, I judge no one but if I judge, my judgement will be sound because I am not alone; the one who sent me is with me:'(5)

Here as in other passages there is a certainty which in any other circumstances could be interpreted as arrogance, delusion or imagination. But the certainty never varies.

> 'If God were your father, you would love me, since I have come here from God. Yes, I have come from him'.[6]

and again

> 'The Father and I are one'[7]

or

> 'The Father is in me and I am in the Father'[8]

In this closeness there is the certainty of unconditional acceptance, the essential prerequisite for the secure growth and development of every person.

> 'If I were to seek my own glory
> that would be no glory at all
> My glory is conferred by the Father'[9]
> 'As the Father has loved me,
> so I have loved you'[10]
> 'I tell you most solemnly anything you ask for
> from the Father he will grant in my name'[11]

These and other passages indicate Christ's utter confidence that his father acknowledged, approved and accepted him without qualification. He had been chosen to carry out a mission, to reconcile man to the Father. He loved the Father and he loved man and because of this love he chose freely the incarnation and the cross. But in undertaking this tremendous task he was supported by a self knowledge which could not be daunted by any human circumstances.

> 'It is true that I am testifying on your behalf
> but my testimony is still valid,
> because I know
> where I came from and where I am going'[12]

When the Jews became utterly impatient and sarcastic the reply is devastating.

> 'My glory is conferred by the Father
> by the one of whom you say 'He is our God'
> although you do not know him.
> But I know him and if I were to say I do not know him
> I should be a liar, as you are liars yourselves.

But I do know him and I faithfully keep his word.
Your father Abraham rejoiced to think he could
see my Day he saw it and was glad.'

The Jews then said 'You are not fifty yet, and
you have seen Abraham!'

Jesus replied

'I tell you most solemnly before Abraham ever was
I am'[13]

Psychologically this last sentence is breathtaking. The passage
of time, change and the various facets of disintegration have no
impact in this unique personality. 'Before Abraham ever was I
am' carries us into a concept of continuing and unchangeable identity beyond any circumscribed human experience and an overwhelming protection against the threat of death. It is of the utmost
significance to note that this categorical assertion of personal
permanency is linked in this passage with the relationship to the
Father. So long as Christ felt close to the Father, no threat existed
to his identity and he encountered no difficulty in facing his approaching death. But his feelings of closeness were so threatened twice.
I use the word feelings here purposely. Both in the Garden of
Gethsemane and on the cross Christ experienced extreme emotional
disturbance. Mark refers to 'sudden fear' and great distress.
Matthew writes about sadness and distress and Luke describes his
anguish and the sweat that fell to the ground like great drops of
blood. All these descriptions in the garden are characteristic of
an anxiety crisis with acute somatic manifestations and a marked
mood swing towards depression. These are exactly the manifestations experienced by the patients who have morbid preoccupation
with death and fear personal dissolution. In Our Lord's case these
symptoms emerge at the moment when there is a crisis of his
identity and a threatened separation between himself and the Father.
If he was to remain the person he was, he had to go on and meet his
death however terrifying this prospect might suddenly have become
to him. To do otherwise would have disrupted the links with the
father. This was not possible and intellectually he knew this. In
John's gospel, Christ praying to the Father at about the same time
asserts unequivocally:-

'Father, may they be one in us
as you are in me and I am in you'[14]

Intellectual certainty that he and the Father are one and the mission
entrusted to him could not be denied, nevertheless did not stop the
emotional upheaval. This dichotomy between intellect and the will
on the one hand and the emotions on the other is a recurrent feature of psychiatric work and demonstrates the absolute need to get
away from the view held for so long which laid the emphasis on the
intellectual and conative aspects of the human personality. There
is abundant evidence to relate the emotional integrity of the individual with both the environment of his upbringing and his inheritance.
As far as the environment is concerned the threat of displeasure
and consequent separation from the beloved parent is a source of
great upheaval amply demonstrated by Christ who while he knew
he could not let his Father down, experienced one of his two episodes of acute emotional distress at the moment this became a
possibility.

Christ, however, possessed such strong bonds with the Father,
that he was able to overcome the fear and to continue in his role.
The security of his relationship with the Father overcame the dread
of personal disintegration and he continued with his passion.

> 'Father', he said, 'If you are willing, take
> this cup away from me. Nevertheless, let
> your will be done, not mine.[15]

The Father's will led to the cross where the second episode of
crisis is encountered.

In Matthew's and Mark's gospels we have identical references.

> 'Eli, Eli, Lama Sabachthani,
> that is 'My God, my God, why have you
> deserted me?'[16]

The whole of Our Lord's identity depended, as the scriptures demonstrate beyond any shadow of doubt, on his indissoluble union of love
with the Father. The feeling of desertion, of abandonment expressed
by Christ on the cross, is in my opinion the most painful moment of
Our Lord's life. Closeness with the father was the guarantee of his
existence and at that moment Christ experienced aloneness and
with it the excruciating agony of isolation. The relevance for the
human personality needs no further elaboration from me. But
Christ's last experience was not that of abandonment.

> 'Father into your hands I commit my spirit'
> With these words he breathed his last.[17]

The words 'Into your hands I commit my spirit' come from Psalm
31.

> 'Pull me out of the net they have spread for me,
> for you are my refuge;
> into your hands I commit my spirit
> You have redeemed me, Yahweh'[18]

Our Lord dies with the certainty of the unuttered sentence, fulfilled
in his Father.

All Christians are involved in the threefold process of creation,
salvation and eschatological fulfilment and for the completion of the
circle death is an inescapable reality. Only through death can we
join in the triumph of the resurrection. But the life of faith has to
be built on the natural order, where pain, suffering, distress are
concrete experiences. The Christian pre-occupation with death
stands in marked contrast to an age which is consciously preoccupied with minimising by every possible means this reality. This
is understandable in terms of a philosophy of life that will not
entertain existence beyond the here and now. Perhaps nowhere
else than at death's door does humanism and Christianity part
their ways so completely. For the humanist death leaves behind
a physical, social and cultural contribution which allows the con-
tinuity of the race physically and aesthetically. For the Christian
death leaves behind all this but adds the Kingdom of God. Christianity has rightly emphasised the need to assist and comfort the
dying and to inspire them at these critical moments with the hope
and courage that will sustain their faith. The care of the dying is
a field in which contemporary Christianity has a lot to contribute
in this country and we owe much to the work of Dr. C. Saunders
and all those who assist her. This is a task which we must continue and extend.

But as you may have guessed I want to conclude with a different
concept. It would seem to me that preparation for death does not
only need the right circumstances to support those about to face
this event but also the promotion of an identity which allows the
personality to anticipate it with the equanimity of Christ. Preparation for death starts with the right human environment in which
personality can grow securely, with the fullest possible self acceptance and a purposeful sense of direction. Only in the fullness of
being human can death find an acceptance which minimises its
stress. For this Christianity needs to complement its work at the
time of death with attention at the time of birth and the early years
of development in the family. The last half century has opened for

us unparalleled avenues in which psychology has given us remarkable insights about the integrity of the human personality. It has
to be admitted sadly that Christianity has been desperately slow
to seize the opportunities that have now been opened to us. The
tools are there for further work and research to deepen our understanding of the best conditions under which the growth of an identity
should take place. Christianity must become involved at both ends
of life so that journey's end is accomplished with the sense of
accomplishment that we see on the Cross. Death will always remain a threat to us but our ability to overcome it will depend on
our ability to develop intact human personalities on which the life
of faith and grace will have the maximum impact. Such thorough
integration is seen in the life and approach to death of Christ. We
have reached a point in history when we can make further use of
the abundance of love that His life and example have given to us.

REFERENCES

1. Luke 2 : 48-50
2. Luke 8 : 21
3. Matthew 3 : 17 (R.S.V.)
4. John 6 : 57
5. John 8 : 15-16
6. John 8 : 42
7. John 10 : 30
8. John 10 : 38
9. John 8 : 54
10. John 15 : 9
11. John 16 : 23
12. John 8 : 14
13. John 8 : 54 : 58
14. John 17 : 21
15. Luke 22 : 43
16. Matthew 27 : 46-47; Mark 15 : 34
17. Luke 23 : 46
18. Psalm 31 : 4-5

BEREAVEMENT

WITH PARTICULAR REFERENCE TO ITS MEDICAL REPERCUSSIONS

C. Murray Parkes

Psychiatrists traditionally study mental illness. Most mental illnesses are presumed to arise from interaction between the society in which we live and the individuals who live in it. Inevitably, we find, when we come to investigate a particular mental illness, a case of alcoholism, for example, that there are many antecedent events which seem in one way or another to have contributed to the person's breakdown. In writing about bereavement as a cause of mental ill health, I do not mean to imply that it is a unitary cause; that patients who break down following bereavement are breaking down simply and solely because of the bereavement. In the past, the tendency among psychiatrists, for obvious reasons, was to start with a sick patient and to try to work back to the cause of the sickness. Hence we made studies of the causes of alcoholism, the causes of schizophrenia, and so on, and ended up with a rag-bag of congenital and environmental causes for these conditions. We found it very difficult to evaluate these and to decide in an individual case how much each of these factors had contributed to the final outcome.

The approach to the problem described here comes from a rather different direction. Instead of starting with an 'illness' and seeking its cause I have started with a particular stress and tried to discover how people cope with it; both those who go on to develop some physical or mental illness and those who go on to make a satisfactory adjustment. (Possibly even a better adjustment than they had prior to the stress.) Because it is a psychiatrist who is writing about bereavement do not get the idea that the effects are necessarily baneful. Not everyone who is bereaved is a serious mental health risk.

The normal or typical reaction to bereavement is grief. By grief I mean the reaction to loss. Most of the stresses that are commonly regarded as potential dangers to health involve either a loss or a threat of loss. Bereavements are particularly severe

stresses. They are common, but they do not occur commonly in
the lives of any one of us: they tend to be scattered throughout life
and to occur relatively infrequently to particular individuals. However, grief is not the only problem to be considered; we have to
remember that someone who has suffered a loss is likely to go on
suffering the deprivation of the person who has been lost and all
the functions previously performed by that person. For instance,
a woman who loses her husband not only loses her husband, she loses
the money and possessions that went with him. The majority of
widows undergo a severe drop in income. They no longer have their
husband's companionship, no longer have the opportunity of sexual
relationships and so on. This, I think, is reflected in their adjustment
in both long and short term.

The bereaved person also undergoes major changes in her roles.
The roles of a widow in our society are different from the roles of
a married woman. There is very often a widow sub-culture, another
society, whose existence the widow may hardly have recognised
prior to her bereavement. This new society exists and she has to
learn to live in it. She has to learn to be a widow. She is also a
survivor. There is a sense in which when someone close to us dies
our own survival becomes a matter of question. As long as we go
through life without losing someone close to us we can pretend that
the world is a safe secure place. When someone close to us dies we
become aware that this kind of thing can happen and if it could happen
to somebody else close to us, it can happen to us. The fact that it
has happened to them and not to us, in some sense, puts us in their
debt. This, of course, is particularly conspicuous when you have
disasters affecting large numbers of people. An important study
by Robert Lifton, [1] of the survivors of the Hiroshima bomb, describes the communal guilt among the survivors. 'Guilt', says Lifton
'is immediately stimulated by participation in the breakdown of the
general human order and by separation from it.'

Then, of course, there are the other roles which have to be taken
up to replace the person who died; for instance, the role of bread-
winner is commonly the widow's role from now on. So we have
grief, deprivation, role change and finally stigma. In any society
there are several value systems that determine how people in that
society are placed in the social hierarchy. In our society a married
woman has, at most times, a higher status than an unmarried woman
or a widow. Furthermore, a woman who loses her husband is an
object of pity; and pity is a very belittling thing. This is something
of which widows complain a great deal: how everybody is sorry for
them. I think the reason they complain is the feeling that they are

somehow being made objects of charity, looked down upon by the
very people who, with all their kindness and sympathy, are trying
to help: but they are trying to help in quite the wrong way.

A lot of people are very much embarrassed and frightened by
the bereaved. They will avoid visiting friends who have been bereaved, and widows will tell you that there were certain people who
did not come near after the bereavement; 'You find out who your
friends are,' they say. An interesting study by Cochrane compares
the way in which different societies treat widows. In many societies
there is quite clearly a strong taboo placed upon the widow, who is
regarded as a very dangerous person. In one society in the Philip-
pines, for instance, no one is allowed to come near the widow. It is
believed that if they do come near her there is a danger of their
becoming sick and dying. Wherever the widow goes she taps on the
trees to warn people of her coming, and it is believed that even the
trees which she taps on will die. So quite clearly the widow is
caught up in the stigma of death and has become an object of danger.
I suspect that something of this fear persists at an unconscious
level in our society.

Let us now consider how unselected widows in London react to
bereavement. I interviewed a group of 22 unselected London widows,
under the age of 65, a month after bereavement and then at three
monthly intervals throughout their first year of bereavement. I was
told of these widows by their general practitioners who had been
asked to refer all newly bereaved widows to me and not only those
who had problems. Nineteen of these 22 widows had been told of
the seriousness of their husband's illness prior to his death, but
only six had fully accepted this. They tended either to deny the
diagnosis or, more commonly, to accept that the doctor's diagnosis
was correct but to deny the prognosis assuming that their husband
was not really going to die or that he would live for much longer
than the doctor indicated. When the husband did finally die, the
immediate reaction in about half the cases was a feeling of numbness
or blunting and I regard this as the first stage of the reaction to
bereavement. It has been described in various studies of the reactions to stress, particularly major disasters and has sometimes
been called the stage of shock. It is described by widows as a feeling
of blunting or numbness— 'I couldn't feel anything, I didn't really
take it in.' This lasts for a few hours to a few days, very seldom
for more than a fortnight, and it is then that the pangs of grief begin.
The characteristic feature of the pang of grief is episodes of intense
pining for the lost person. John Bowlby who has written about reactions to loss in childhood, has called this the stage of yearning

and protest. [2] These intense episodes of pining are associated with
subjective psychic pain and autonomic (under unconscious nervous
control) disturbance, sweating, deep sighing respiration, palpitations
very often, dryness in the mouth, the kinds of phenomenon which one
associates with stimulation of the sympathetic nervous system. The
widow is very restless and preoccupied with thoughts of loss and of
the lost person. Pangs are precipitated by any reminder of the loss
and in between times there is a feeling of apathy, with episodes of
restlessness and, as one widow put it, 'continually searching for
something to do but unable to carry out any activity to its finish'.
At this time one also finds a change in perceptual set, such that the
lost person is felt to be near at hand. Fifteen out of the 22 widows
described a strong sense of the presence of the dead person. As
one said, 'I can almost feel his skin and touch his hands'.

In this series there were nine widows who described actual
illusions of the presence of the dead person. One widow described
how she was walking down the street and saw her husband coming
towards her, then as he got closer she realized she was mistaken.
This kind of thing is commonly reported. A click may be misinter-
preted as the husband's key in the lock and hypnagoguic (occurring
during sleep) hallucinations, as they are called, may occur. One
woman described how she was sitting resting in a chair in the garden
and she thought she saw her husband digging with his shirt off, quite
vividly.

Many of these symptoms can be understood as a suppression of
an urge to search for the lost person. [3] If we think of the way in
which animals react to loss—the pining, the intense searching, and
crying aloud for a lost cub or another member of the herd—there is
obviously a parallel here. For some widows, there is a recognition
of this. Widows have told me: 'I walk around searching for him';
'I felt that if I had gone somewhere I would have found him'; 'I go to
the grave but he's not there'; 'I am just searching for nothing'.
Darwin, in 'The Expression of the Emotions in Man and Animals'
has suggested that the expression of sorrow is a suppressed form
of the behaviour which we see in unrestrained form in young children who are crying for their mother. The sob is thus a suppressed
cry as are the drawing down of the corners of the mouth and the
screwing up of the eyes.

There are both inhibitory factors and factors trying to press
towards expression of emotion. Thus the bereaved person is in a
state of conflict and will oscillate between being pulled towards a
place associated with the dead person and avoiding it. For example,
one widow I talked to had repeatedly moved from the front bedroom

where she slept with her husband to the back bedroom in an effort to avoid the pangs of grief, but when she was in the back bedroom, she felt drawn back to the front bedroom because somehow she would be closer to him there; you can see the ambivalence involved in this. Some of this attempt to avoid reminders is conscious, some of it is perhaps unconscious. The widow will often say, 'I still can't really believe that it's true'. She has difficulty in accepting the fact of loss.

As time passes the pangs of grief gradually diminish and the periods of apathy and depression become more marked. There is no sharp transition between the stage of yearning and the third stage, the stage of despair. The period of numbness is succeeded by spikes of intense grieving and eventually these gradually diminish in frequency and severity. But I do not think we can say that there is a clear end to grieving. Even years after a major loss, an anniversary or a reminder, finding a photograph in a drawer, can precipitate again episodes of severe pining. As the intense pining diminishes periods of despair and aimlessness supervene and these in turn are followed by the final stage or reorganization, when the widow gradually takes up again her interests in life, her appetite returns (she has lost a stone or two in weight), and within three or four months she is beginning to pick up weight. Other interests gradually revive, sleeping gradually gets better but rather less quickly than return of appetite for food. I think the emphasis on reorganisation here is important in that to a large extent the bereaved person has lost a whole set of expectations and assumptions about life; her world has got to be organized afresh and it is in this phase that she sets about the task of reorganisation.

I come now to the pathological consequences of bereavement. First of all, what evidence have we that bereavement can have pathological consequences? I was able to study the case notes of 44 unselected widows registered with their GPs two years before and after bereavement.[4] The widows were not selected, the GPs were; they were selected on the grounds that they had helped us with previous research and we knew that these particular GPs kept exceptionally good case records. I stress this because GP case records are not the best source of research data. Let us first consider the GP consultation rate among 29 widows under the age of 65, during six month periods before and after bereavement. This study showed that there was a sharp increase in the consultation rate during the first six months, which was maintained at a slightly lower level during the second and third six month periods. We were not able to follow these widows up beyond this time. As I think you would expect,

the greatest increase was for symptoms which we called psychiatric.
They included attendances for depression, insomnia or any condition
treated with sedative or similar drug.

In the over 65 age group, however, this was not the case. There
were fifteen patients who also showed an increase in consultations
for pyschiatric symptoms. Whereas in the under 65 age group there
was a sevenfold increase in sedative prescriptions in the first six
months, maintained, but at a lower level, during the next year; in
the over 65 age group there was very little change in sedative prescriptions.

Turning to another source of information about the consequences
of bereavement, I studied the incidence of loss of spouse in psychiatric patients attending the Bethlem and Maudsley Hospitals.[5]
Here I was trying to find out how many patients admitted to the
Bethlem and Maudsley Hospitals had lost a spouse during the six
months prior to the onset of their presenting illness. And in fact
the incidence was six times greater than one would have expected
had this group had the same mortality rate as the population as a
whole. Using the Registrar General's figures, one was able to estimate
how many patients one would have expected to be admitted during
that period if there had been a chance relationship between the
bereavement and the mental illness.

Another source of data is the study of mortality rates. In 1963
Young, Benjamin and Wallis, showed that there is an increased mortality rate among widowers over the age of 55 during the first six
months after the wife's death, returning to near the level for married people of the same age during the subsequent two years.[6] More
recently,[7] a further study of these patients has been carried out
which shows this rise in mortality during the first six months after
bereavement is very largely attributable to death from heart disease
particularly coronary thrombosis. Various theories have been put
forward to account for this finding but there is no space to discuss
them here. It is worth reflecting, however, that perhaps, the old
notion that you can die of a broken heart is not such a medical myth
as it has been thought to be.

Let us go on now to look more closely at other illnesses that
follow bereavement. There have been many studies of conditions
such as ulcerative colitis (inflammatory disease of the bowel)
asthma, rheumatoid arthritis, and even leukaemia, claiming relationships between bereavement and these illnesses, again there is not
space to discuss them here. Despite considerable difficulties in
researching this field I think there is good reason for believing that
many psychosomatic conditions may be precipitated by bereavement.

When we come to look at psychological complaints, there have been studies showing a relationship between, for instance, alcoholism and bereavement. This is hardly surprising since we might expect that someone who has been a heavy drinker all his life will drink more heavily when his wife dies. Less easy to explain are cases of acute mania coming on following bereavement. There are over fourteen of these described in the literature, and I have come across one, where the onset of the mania did coincide with the bereavement very closely. In most of the accounts in the literature and the cases that I have seen one of the striking features was the way in which the manic patient denied the reality of his loss. In one way or another, he went on behaving as if the dead person was still alive.

The commonest form of psychological disturbances after bereavement, is the pathological grief reaction. In a study of 21 bereaved psychiatric patients, I found that in 20 cases there was reason to believe that the grief for the loss was in some way or another abnormal. Two major kinds of pathological reaction were apparent. The first of these has been called 'chronic grief'. This syndrome was first described by Anderson, [8] and it occurred in 15 out of my 21 bereaved psychiatric patients. These were still showing all the signs of acute grief 6 months or more after the death of their relative. Their grief showed very little sign of abating years later. The other main type of reaction was what has been called 'delayed grief'. There were 8 people who had reacted in this way in my series—these were people who had shown very little emotion at the time of the loss and then broken down much later. You will recall that the period of numbness seldom continues for more than a fortnight. In all of these psychiatric patients either the stage of numbness persisted or they denied even feeling numb. In this study and in others it does appear that those people who delay the onset of their grief are the ones who subsequently become most disturbed.

Although I have divided up these pathological grief reactions into chronic and delayed patterns, I do not think it is an important distinction. I think that once the grief does emerge, it tends to take a rather similar pattern whether it comes on at once or is delayed. There are other features which were found in my bereaved psychiatric patients much more commonly than in the unselected widows whom I described earlier. Six of my 21 psychiatric patients were suffering from panic attacks, these were particularly likely to come on at a time when the husband would be arriving home from work. These could be very alarming and disruptive. Five patients had hypochondriacal illnesses, closely resembling the illness the husband had had during his terminal disease. For instance, one man was admitted to hospital with what appeared to be a coronary thrombosis, typical coronary pain. He was referred to a psychiatrist when investigation of his heart function proved normal, and subsequently in psychotherapy, he made the link between his 'coronary' symptoms and the illness which his father had suffered. He got better, was discharged and a few weeks later he was back again, this time with an abdominal pain. This pain closely resembled another symptom which his father had had during his final illness.

The other psychological reaction which was very common in the psychiatric group was expression of intense guilt and self-blame. It is common enough for bereaved people to go over in their minds the events leading up to the death in an attempt to find some cause for the death. People often seize on some minor omission and blame themselves for it. But in the bereaved psychiatric patient this was much more likely to be a major preoccupation. In both cases the expression of guilt was very often illogical and unrealistic.

Why do some people break down after bereavements whilst others remain well-adjusted? The research into this question has not yet been very satisfactory. When you have many different causes contributing to a particular outcome it is hard to pin down the ones that are most important. From now on I shall be writing from clinical experience of working with bereaved people rather than from careful systematic studies based on statistical findings. My impression is that there are three main areas to be borne in mind in considering the psychopathology of pathological grief. The nature of the loss, the way in which the bereaved person copes with it, and the help which he gets from others. First of all, let us look at the magnitude and nature of the loss. Where, for instance, there has been a highly dependent relationship with the dead husband, as you might expect, the surviving widow is going to have a big problem adjusting to life without him. It does not have to be the widow who is herself dependent on her husband, it can be the other way round. It may be that a woman has for many years looked after her husband and he has been highly dependent on her. When he dies she is left without a 'baby', she has lost a whole major role in her life and adjustment may be very difficult.

Then there are marriages where there is a highly ambivalent relationship. People who have for years been fighting, quarrelling, leaving one another. I saw one widow who said, a week after her husband's death—'Well, quite frankly I am glad to be rid of him, I left him many times, he gambled all the housekeeping money away, he used to drink like a fish,' and so on. A year later, she was deeply depressed. She said, 'If I could find another man just like my hus-

band I would marry him tomorrow.' Sudden unexpected losses seem
to provoke more severe reactions as you might expect than losses
that have come over a gradual period when the survivor has had a
chance to prepare herself for what is coming.

The second major type of factor determining the reaction to
bereavement is those things that influence the means of coping with
grief. People who do not break down, who defend themselves against
grief—perhaps there is a family tradition to keep a stiff upper lip—
commonly have delayed reactions. In our society there is a tendency
for us to take less and less account of the rituals associated with
mourning. Geoffrey Gorer has written a fully documented account of
mourning behaviour in Britain today[9] and he believes that many of
the pathological reactions that we see are attributable to a culture
which does not permit the free expression of emotion. I think it is
important to remember that it is not only the sense of pining and
despair that needs to be expressed but very often feelings of anger,
bitterness and resentment. Many people find it more difficult to
admit that they feel bitter and angry at what has happened than to
admit that they feel sad.

The third type of factor which influences outcome following bereavement, is the social environment. Widows who are socially isolated, particularly women without children, seem less likely to make
a satisfactory adjustment. On the other hand, widows who have an
over-protective family may also do badly. Occasionally one comes
across the type of reaction exemplified by Queen Victoria, where
the memory of the dead husband has to be kept alive, and everybody
in the family is expected to call on the widow and pay tribute. At
the time when Victoria died she was still having Albert's nightgown
laid out on the bed each night and hot water put out for him. Geoffrey
Gorer calls this process 'fossilisation'. I think this is one of those
areas where it is possible for psychiatrists to give help by support-
ing the front line workers, as Gerald Caplan has termed them. That
is to say, the clergy, general practitioners, social workers and
relatives who are in daily contact with people who are undergoing
the experience of bereavement. They can often do more good by
acting as consultants to these people than they can by actually working with bereaved people. I am not saying they should not offer
direct help to bereaved people, but that there are two possible roles
for them here. Whilst it would obviously be impossible for a psychiatrist to see every woman who loses her husband, every husband
who loses his wife, every child who loses a parent and so on, nevertheless, there are people in the care-giving professions who do and
will in the course of their everyday work meet these people.

There is no specific treatment which will allay grief. Grief, it seems, must be suffered if the survivor is to adjust to life without the dead person. The task of the care-giver, therefore, is to try to ensure that conditions make it possible for the bereaved person to grieve, to reassure him of the normality of the strange and often frightening feelings and thoughts which he experiences and, when the peak of grief is past, to point the way towards a more realistic and satisfying adjustment to life.

REFERENCES

1. Lifton, R. J. *Death in Life: The Survivors of Hiroshima.* Weidenfeld & Nicholson, 1968.

2. Bowlby, J., 'Processes of Mourning' in International Journal of Psychoanalysis, 1962, p. 62 and 317.

3. Evidence for this hypothesis is given in my paper 'Separation Anxiety: An Aspect of the Search for a Lost Object', published in *Studies in Anxiety,* Ed. M. H. Lader, Headley Bros., 1969.

4. Parkes, C. M. Brit. Med. J. 1964, 2: 274.

5. Parkes, C. M. *British Journal of Psychiatry* 1964, **110**: 198

6. *Lancet,* 2: 454.

7. Parkes, C. M., Benjamin, B. and Fitzgerald, R. C. *British Medical Journal* 1969, **1**: 740.

8. International Journal of Psychoanalysis 1949, **30**: 48.

9. *Death, Grief and Mourning in Contemporary Britain.* Cresset, 1965.

ORGAN TRANSPLANTATION

R. Calne

This subject is a matter of great controversy and public interest
and it was inflamed in every newspaper a few months ago to a degree
unprecedented, I believe, in any medical activity in the past. The
publicity that followed transplantation of the heart threw everything
out of perspective and caused much disquiet. Now the public and
the profession are beginning to swing back into a more even keel
and are considering what is really quite a straightforward and simple advance in medical treatment.

The object of organ transplantation is no different from the object of any other kind of medical or surgical therapy. It is to try to
restore somebody who is afflicted with a fatal illness, to a happy
and useful life. The only difference from other types of therapy is
that one is considering disease of a vital organ whose function must
be replaced; otherwise the patient will die. An organ such as the
appendix can have a life-threatening disease, acute appendicitis,
where the treatment to save the patient's life and to restore him to
a happy and healthy existence is merely to remove the appendix.
You cannot do that with the liver and the heart, or with diseases
affecting both kidneys. The function of these organs must be restored. There are only two ways available to do this; one is to con-
struct an artificial, mechanical and chemical prosthesis, and the
other is to replace the missing function by a biologically active
graft. This is the *raison d'être* of transplantation surgery; it is very
simple and the way in which it needs to be fulfilled does not need to
interfere with any traditional medical ethics.

I think it is very unfortunate that the contrary opinion has been
expressed, usually by people who have no experience of transplantation and who have no responsible background in the field. The heart,
which is the source of this tremendous publicity, is simply a pump;
it is a very fine pump with its own built-in motor and source of
energy, but it is nothing more. It seems that most people refuse to
accept this fact, probably because the heart beats fast at times of
emotion and because absence of the heartbeat is the traditionally
accepted method of diagnosing death. Also, of course, because for
thousands of years the heart has been invested with emotions of
love. Nevertheless, it is a pump and if one could produce a good

mechanical substitute it ought to be able to do the function of the heart; one day probably this will be achieved. At the moment the engineers are behind the transplanters in this respect.

The liver is a much more complicated organ. We don't know more than a fragment of its functions, so there is no possibility in the foreseeable future of replacing its actions artificially; one has to graft a liver to save a patient suffering from irreversible liver disease. The kidney is somewhere in between. We can cope with most of the kidney functions artificially; the apparatus required to do it is rather cumbersome and has certain disadvantages.

There are occasions where it is justifiable for live donors to give a kidney for transplantation. They should preferably be closely related to the recipient, for example a parent giving a kidney to a child. This circumstance does not arise very often in the United Kingdom, although it seems to be rather more common in the United States. Out of 70 kidney transplants performed in Cambridge only three have been from live donors, all of whom were parents. With regard to animal donors—one day we hope that animals will provide suitable organs for transplantation to men and there is much work being devoted to the immunology of heterografts. It is unlikely that there will be much success in this field until the results of man to man grafting are uniformly successful.

I will finish by saying a few words about cadaveric donors, because this is where my main experience lies. As far as the public is concerned I think there are only three factors of reassurance required to establish that this is an ethical procedure.

First of all they must be dead and there must have been no interference with their care prior to death directed towards transplantation. Secondly, the organ must be used for a good purpose or an attempt must be made to use the organ for a good purpose in good faith. Thirdly, the privacy of the bereaved next of kin will not be invaded and blazened across newspapers in the shameful way that has happened with some of the heart transplant relatives—pictures of honeymoon couples and of bereaved aged parents coming to the funeral of the person who died. I think this has been one of the most distasteful aspects of recent publicity; it has done a great deal of harm to the image of the idea of transplantation.

I maintain the diagnosis of death is not difficult. Most lay people can diagnose death, certainly most nurses, and if a doctor cannot diagnose death he should not be a doctor. There are cases where it may be a little difficult to be sure that the patient is dead; under such circumstances the course is obvious to the doctor—to regard the patient as alive until he has no doubt that the patient is dead.

Traditional methods of diagnosing death are perfectly adequate for transplantation, namely cessation of heartbeat and cessation of respiration. Any decision to stop resuscitation should be quite independent of transplantation considerations. The decision is made in good faith towards the patient who is being treated and his relatives, and not in relation to possible transplantation; there is no need why this should be changed. If the doctor feels that he has done his very best and there is no hope of independent existence for his patient, then resuscitation is usually stopped. This has been an accepted medical procedure years before transplantation was thought of. The Pope has recently made a statement on this point saying that it is not incumbent upon a medical man to use extraordinary means to maintain life. I think this fits in with traditional medical ethics.

Organs deteriorate rapidly after death, the liver is more sensitive than the heart and the heart more so than the kidney, yet it is possible to get excellent function from a transplanted liver that has been taken from a patient who has not been touched until death has been diagnosed by conventional means. Since this is possible there seems to be no reason to tamper with the diagnosis of death. There is no point in changing the diagnosis of death if what is accepted and has been accepted for thousands of years, is sufficient to transplant and get excellent function from the most sensitive organ that one needs to transplant. I feel that these principles should be made known, not only in the medical and nursing professions but also to the public.

There is a very important ethical problem in transplantation that has received much less attention than it should. In this country every year between two and three thousand young people are dying of kidney disease and less than two hundred of these are getting any offer of treatment. Yet we know that even with the traditional methods of immuno-suppression and without tissue typing, using random cadaver donors, it is possible to have 50% of these patients leading a normal or nearly normal life a year later and almost 50% at two years. With transplants from close blood-relations the results are even better. Now, techniques of immuno-suppression and tissue typing are improving, and I think that the profession and the public need to look very seriously as to whether we can afford to allow all these people to die unnecessarily. Organ transplantation is becoming cheaper, restoration of a chronically sick person back to work is of economic benefit to the country. The cost, in any case, is irrelevant in terms of the vast billions spent on fighting planes that never even fly—let alone fight.

I have said enough. As you can see, there is only one problem, namely we are not transplanting enough organs, since the demand greatly exceeds the supply. If we lower the emotional tone and comply with traditional medical ethics, there is no reason why transplantation should not become a routine part of modern therapeutic surgery.

THE DONOR CRISIS IN ORGAN TRANSPLANTATION

W. J. Dempster

The crisis in organ donors is not an isolated phenomenon in medicine as a whole today. For some time there has been a smouldering debate about motivation in medicine. There are those who consider it right to prolong life even when its quality is poor. On the other hand there is increasing unease about the inhumanity which can result from such a policy. There are those who believe that the judgement of many doctors is becoming too subservient to the tyranny of their skills which enable them to maintain life artificially without the quality necessary for human happiness. Should therapeutic intervention be an unqualified rule in the practice of clinical medicine? Is there any virtue in maintaining some bodily functions artificially with machines, when the ability to appreciate and recognise one's surroundings has long departed? Organ transplantation as we know it today, fits into this general problem.

The crisis of donors for organ transplantation is really part of the wider issue of deciding which patients are to be provided with artificial respiration and when the machines are to be switched off. This is the real crisis and medical opinion is divided about it. Some patients are kept on the respirators for a few hours, whilst others are maintained for years in the hope that recovery may eventually occur. The decisions inevitably depend to some extent on the type of hospital and on the interests and skills available, but careful assessment is required in reaching conclusions about the criteria for recognition of the irrecoverable state. Even then one must consider in whose best interests any further therapeutic measures are carried out. Vested interests, medico-legal issues, technical prestige and motivation directed solely to the welfare of the patients are all involved in arriving at decisions, so that discussion about the ethics of this aspect of medicine can become a sterile and invidious argument. The general public provides the finance for hospitals and the health service, and increasingly demands to be informed about modern trends in medicine. No longer can the physician hope to be his own counsel, jury and judge of whether a clinical experiment is justifiable.

Within ten years of the Nuremburg war trials, directives had to
be sent to medical clinics in this country setting limits on the kind
of experiments which could justifiably be carried out on patients in
the course of research. With the best of intentions doctors had gone
beyond what many other doctors considered humanitarian. The conflict between extracting scientific data by experiment and the rights
of the patient is an old one. Claude Bernard, writing a century ago,
arrived at this conclusion: 'The principle of medical morality con-
sists, then, in never performing on man an experiment which can be
harmful to him in any degree whatsoever though the results may be
of great interest to science—that is of benefit to save the health of
others'. In recent years, further directives have been issued to
medical clinics defining more clearly the conditions under which
experiments may be carried out. Clearly earlier directives were
not being respected by a sufficient number of doctors. All advanced
countries are faced with the same predicament and we have experiences in other aspects of human endeavour that the road to hell
can be paved with good intentions.

The dilemma evoked by the conflicting demands of the individual,
his team and the public as patients must lie in creating trust and
confidence based on clear information. Is one to do nothing, then,
to help desperately ill patients? To do nothing is frequently a positive judgement in the best interests of the patient as a human being.
To prolong life by some major procedure may mean no more than a
few days of further discomfort and the raising of false hopes in the
relatives. All medical advances have had their human guinea pigs
and failures. What the public should be informed about is that, no
matter how many organs are transplanted with the techniques available now, the results will improve only marginally. Similarly, the
rate of cure in many forms of cancer, treated by modern techniques,
will not improve.

How far is the public prepared to go with organ transplants?
It has indicated that, so far as abortion is concerned, it is prepared
to go a good deal further than the medical profession and it would
appear that the public is not as squeamish as some may think. The
indications are that the majority of people want organ transplants
and want to know the facts about the scientific necessities underlying
a donor service.

If organ transplantation is to work in the future, the public,
through Parliament, must decide the legal issues on which it depends.
In readjusting our official ethics to meet the current scientific
necessities, a section of the community will suffer moral and spiritual agony. This is inevitable, but some of us suffer agony as the
law stands now.

In what way do we have to arrange our ethics so that the ac-
credited moral values are in harmony with the scientific necessities?
It is essential that the medical and lay public should know what
alternative sources of organs are available for transplantations.
These are:

1. The healthy volunteer donor: This source is limited to the
    kidney but many transplanters object to it even here and believe
    that the issue should never be presented to the interested
    parties.

2. The hopeless respirator cases: These, by private agreement
    throughout the world, are being subjected to removal of organs
    before and immediately after the respirator is switched off.
    Such organs are classified as 'cadaver' and the results are
    good.

3. Those who have died without respirator aid or respirator aid
    given just before death in order to maintain a reasonable cir-
    culation: Organs from these people are removed in a varying
    state of damage and the functional capacity after transplantation
    varies considerably.

4. Animal sources other than man: The interspecies immune re-
    action is so severe that a solution is not yet in sight.

The law requires no adjustment for sources 1 and 4 but the
second and third sources provide moral and legal disputes. The
second source is by far the most scientifically desirable source of
organs for transplantation. Indeed, for heart and liver transplantation it is obligatory. The operation can be planned and many of the
limitations of emergency surgery can be avoided. The Renal Transplantation Bill, proposed by Sir Gerald Nabarro, sought to legalise
the removal of kidneys once a person is declared dead unless the
deceased has instructed otherwise. But, so far as the hopeless respirator case is concerned, we have still not solved or even attempted
to solve legally how and when the declaration is to be made.

This is the rub and this is where the public should be asked to
consider the scientific facts as well as the moral and emotional
issues. In the history of social change moral values change to suit
new conditions. Will the new Bill, taken at its face value, provide
organs in the most suitable state for transplantation? This answer
is no.

For some time now it has been usual to approach relatives before death and to request sanction to remove kidneys immediately
after death. Administrative action has to be taken before death **and**

in actual practice this means preparing the dying patient in the final hours for immediate nephrectomy (removal of the kidneys) after he dies. Sometimes the dying patient has been prepared for operation in a room adjoining the operating theatre so as to curtail the period of anoxia (lack of oxygen) and consequent damage to the kidneys. Even this degree of anticipation is of little value where hearts and livers are concerned. Bill or no Bill this necessary practice will continue, but it is not clear to everyone that administrative action must be taken before death. This is distasteful to many doctors, but it may be that the public will have no qualms.

Given the choice, it is probable that the public will opt for the respirator donor and will have the good sense to realize quickly that transplantation of severely damaged organs is not in the best interests of the recipients. The rights of the dying donor have been the cause of anxiety in the past but, accepting that the donor is a hopeless case, we must surely now consider the rights of the prospective recipients. The time may even come when the relatives of recipient patients will reserve the right to refuse operation, if the circumstances under which an organ was salvaged inevitably involved moderate to severe damage. Patients should be protected against abuse of organ transplantation by unrealistic enthusiasts trying to make the best of a bad job.

It is, therefore, absurd to introduce 'safeguards' which would seek to exclude the transplant surgeon from the decision to switch off the respirator. Indeed, in formulating any such safeguards, are we really warning the public that an enthusiastic transplanter would end prematurely the life of a hopeless respirator case? Whichever way we care to look at these safeguards, they seem to reflect the nightmarish suspicions of a sick society. The transplanting surgeon must play his part in the collective declaration to end the artificial life of a hopeless respirator case.

However, though the thought of a surgeon who is prepared to end the life of a donor while there is still hope that he will recover, is such anathema that it is repellent even to consider it, the public needs complete reassurance. A new law should specify, therefore, that two neurologists, one of whom should be 'neutral' and from a different hospital, must agree that the point of no return has been reached and that the patient would never recover. Furthermore, doctors should be prepared, so that justice can be seen to be done, to have their records available to appropriate inspection.

The law and our ethics should be adjusted so as to allow realistic transplantation of heart, liver and lungs as well as kidneys. The scientific necessities demand a donor whose circulation is artificially maintained by a respirator and the law should specifically legalize the planned euthanasia of the hopeless respirator case. In whose interest is it to maintain such tragic cases in a state of artificial life until infected lungs end it all? Certainly not in the interests of the dying patient. Certainly not in the interest of the relatives who are subjected to prolonged anguish. At the moment planned euthanasia, by switching off the respirator either before or after the organ has been removed, is carried out by private arrangement and without legal sanction; and the onlooker is powerless.

A THEOLOGIAN'S REFLECTIONS ON SOME AREAS OF SURGICAL PRACTICE

G. R. Dunstan

The theologian shares with the medical man the embarrassment of being the object of conflicting public expectations. The 'progressive', on the one hand, hail every new medical possiblity as an advance, and dismiss in terms of which the word 'conservative' is perhaps the least damning anyone who, on either medical or theological grounds, seems cautious or hesitant about exploiting it. Others, on the other hand, have already drawn a mental line: they are perhaps vague about where, in an historical perspective, they have drawn it, and why precisely there—they would accept, that is to say, the medical ingenuities with which they have grown up, forgetting perhaps the battles by which some of those practices, in their day, became established, but they are cautious about overstepping that line. In the language employed in these circles, doctors who experiment with brain cells, or (even worse) with ova and spermatozoa in test tubes, are interfering with nature; and theologians who will not cry out against them are (as Mr. Muggeridge has said) merely 'slack'; judgement will follow. So we invite suspicion either way, whether we say yes to experimental, exploratory medical science, or whether we say stop.

We are left with a familiar duty, then, to decide our course of action for ourselves, in the light of the general ethical principles, such as they are, enshrined in our respective professional traditions, and then to feel our way, advancing when we think we can and believe we ought to, and holding back when we do not. This does not imply that we should ignore public opinion. That would be bad medical practice, as it would be a bad theological prescription: we live in a time of mounting public protest at being ignored, and an essential step in the ethical refounding of our society must be the engaging of the public in a new sort of social and ethical concern. At the heart of ethics stand expectations—what we commonly expect of one another in recognizably similar situations; and society cannot live very easily for very long with uncertainty in its expectations. So medical ethics, which are first and properly a tradition within the profession of medicine, must be matched by social or public expectations: otherwise there comes a dangerous gap between what the public may demand, and what the ethics of medicine may

permit— or, *vice versa,* between what doctors of a refined, experimental cast of mind may want to do, and what the public will allow
them to do, or at least put up the money for them to do. The
reported statistics about the first nine months of working of the
1968 Abortion Act illustrate the ethical problems of the first sort;
the more sensational aspects of the transplant debate illustrate
those of the second; public fears and emotions have been exploited
to create 'news' and sensational discussion, without regard for considerations integral to the practice.

Public opinion, I said, must not be ignored. It must be educated.
The alternative is exploitation, for it is too valuable a 'market' now
to be left alone. Concerning the ethics of surgical practice, public
opinion is clouded with fear and sentiment. Part of the fear is
understandable, and could be dissolved by good medical practice
and administration, and by a competent use of the mass media to
convince people that they *are* in fact, good. In the transplant debates
the fears are, of course, first that the interests of the donor or
source patient will not be sacrificed to the interests of the recipient
patient; and secondly, that the source patient is already 'dead' (whatever that may now mean), before the organs are taken from him.
Provisions in Sir Gerald Nabarro's recent Renal Transplantation
Bills seemed adequate to cover both concerns; though, had they been
enacted, the task of educating the public to believe in them would
still have remained.

The sentiments are more difficult to handle, for they are more
mixed; and a good deal of vestigial religion, of a sort, is compounded
with them. I propose to give to them what remains of my space, and
I apologise if what I say seems too trivial or too absurd to occupy
your time. For myself, I am surprised to find how often these
trivial things have to be said, precisely because the layers of con-
fusion are so widespread and deep. The sentiments concern the
integrity of the body: what may or may not be done to it without
nefas—an offence to essential proprieties if not to the gods—and its
status *vis à vis* the 'soul', life after death, resurrection or immortality.

These sentiments are deep in man: were they not, the world's
literature, poetry, drama, art, music, would be immeasurably the
poorer. They are not lightly, therefore, to be rationalised or ex-
plained away. In our Western tradition they have clothed themselves
with the language of the Hebrew and Christian scriptures; and since
a literal interpretation of words is more easy both to teach and to
believe than a symbolic interpretation, it is to be expected that
literalism should have imprisoned the imagination and so engendered
fear.

The point is most clearly illustrated in relation to the heart. In the poetry and indeed the common language of romance, the heart is the seat of the affections, of love, of emotional pleasure. Physiologically, I suppose, this is easily understood because of the quickened heart beat when such pleasures intensify. To the literal mind, therefore, when pleasure is no longer speaking its own poetry, to touch the heart is violence indeed. In the Greek and Hebrew traditions these emotional functions were seated in the bowels: and it is only delicacy of a sort which has translated 'bowels' into 'hearts' in our tradition. Religiously, too, literalism has created problems. In the scriptures of the Old and New Testaments the Hebrew and the Greek word translated 'heart' is used *without* physiological reference to denote mind, spirit, soul, will; concentrated attention or devotion; conscience, moral judgement. These writers were not fools: they knew, far more than most of us, the language of symbolism and its power. They would, therefore, have been even more horrified than we are at the language of a clergyman who, a few months ago, publicly opposed heart transplants because the Scripture locates the heart as the dwelling place of Christ. (Ephesians 3: 17). If this can be said by a clergyman, we must expect simple believers to be disturbed. And not simple believers only. There is a wide area of residual Christianity abroad, beyond the frontiers of belief, out of touch with the sources of religious language, and cut off from the religious communities in which that language is always subject to scrutiny and interpretation. In this area, I suspect, the supposed special 'sacredness' or untouchability of the heart is even more deeply entrenched as the focus of sentiment. The primal fear, therefore, the *nefas*, the taboo, can use religious language of a kind, to support itself, to give it a front.

These, I believe, are some of the attitudes which today's surgeon encounters. I have no theological interest in defending them: they are a product of a literalism which can be the worst barrier to religious understanding. But we must understand their attitudes if we are to help people to modify them.

The same must be said about the other group of topics—the relation of 'body' and 'soul', and the language of 'life after death', 'destroying the soul', 'resurrection' or 'immortality'. There is an entirely realistic ambiguity about the body entrenched in the Christian tradition—realistic, I say, because it matches the reality which we know, that the body can be an organ or instrument of bliss, or one of pain, or even one of devilry. Contrary to what is popularly believed, the Christian Church first came into controversy about the body, not to devalue it as against the soul, but to defend the body, to be its champion, against those who sought to exalt the soul by denigrating the body.

The very dualism presupposed in this language of 'soul' and 'body' is, in fact, Platonic in origin, not Christian. St. Paul used— perhaps we may say 'coined'— our contemporary 'psycho-somatic' language; he called the living human organism σῶμα ψυχικόν (I Cor. 15 : 44). For the Platonists the body constituted a tomb or prison from which it is the object of the soul to be free; to achieve this freedom from the body is the aim of philosophy. To quote a recent writer, for the Platonist:

> 'The body is gross, untrustworthy and obtrusive, and detachment from it is to be cultivated as a preparation for death which will bring deliverance from it'. [1]

Against this denigration of the body the early Greek fathers con- tended with vigour. Whenever it appeared—as it did in Manicheeism, and in angelism in various guises—the Church fought it as a heresy. The later weapon was sometimes fire and sword; the earliest weapon was theology, the weapon of minds which had pondered and made some meaning out of the life, death and resurrection of Jesus as the Gospels portrayed it.

The doctrine of the resurrection of the body was evolved and taught precisely to defend this integrity of the body as part of the whole man—an indispensible part, and the handiwork of the one God—the God and father of Jesus Christ. The question of man was inseparable from the question of God: for pagan religion at the time, the God who was concerned with spirit, with 'souls', could not have soiled himself by creating bodies, or anything material at all: that was the work of an anti-God. The dualism about man therefore reflected a dualism about God: and Christian theology tackled both together. Theology affirmed a belief in 'the resurrection of the body' as a defense of the totality of man, as a human being. It did not therby commit itself—as the literalist would seem to suppose—to belief in a resuscitation of all our physical bits and pieces. The Greek fathers could face the question posed, for instance, of a drowned man eaten by fishes or of the man eaten by wild beasts: it simply did not worry them; they were intelligent and learned men. They rested their doctrine on two presuppositions: the first, that man is created 'in God's image', and God, by definition, is incor- poreal, without a body; and secondly that Jesus, when risen from the dead, was (according to the Gospel narratives) seen and recognized, and capable of communication, yet certainly *not* restricted by a material body.

Given these starting points, meaning could express itself only in the language of symbols—of which the language of 'the resurrection of the body' was but a part. These symbols are already in use in St. Paul's letters to the Corinthians, where he can use self-contradictory phrases like 'a spiritual body'—σῶμα ψυχικόν set against σῶμα πνευματικόν and 'a spiritual body' is as telling symbolic language as Milton's 'darkness visible'.

What would a modern theologian say of this? I think he would insist that the language of 'the soul', of 'God's image', and of 'the resurrection of the body' is the language not of concrete physical substance, but of relationship, and of an inalienable capacity for relationship. 'The soul', we might say, is human personality conceived of relationally: in its final analysis towards God: so words like 'the destruction of the soul' could be replaced by the language of 'alienation from God': (McCabe, op. cit. p. 86: 'Having a soul is just being able to communicate; having a mind is being able to communicate linguistically'). The 'integrity of the body' which the modern theologian would defend, therefore, is *not* a supposed completeness of the anatomical parts—the notion becomes absurd, anyhow when one begins to think of the body organically—but the capacity of the body to be an instrument of relationships. To offer a formula like this is by no means to close any question: it is to propose terms in which discussion can begin on such questions as the duty of care owed to a supposedly incurable unconscious patient; or the process and meaning of death. [2] The formula—the language of capacity for relationships—leaves me free, for instance, to see no theological or ethical problem inherent in the transplanting of merely functional organs, like heart, kidney or liver, but to see problems loom around the transplanting of gonads, or of the brain if that became feasible—for these carry some of the constituents of what we call 'personality', and it is 'persons' who 'relate'. It seems to me that we need a formula such as this at least as a basis for discussion of the ethics of these developments if they come—rather than the language of the 'sacredness' of the body, or of this or that part of it, which does not seem to get us very far. (In short, no man's 'soul' or eternal destiny is affected by what a surgeon takes from his body after death; but only by what God, the man himself and society do with him in life—and God alone after life).

I hope I have done no injustice to other men's thoughts, opinions, or sentiments—even to those of an anonymous 'public'. I have drawn only on the Hebrew-Christian tradition, partly because it is the only one which I know much about, and partly because it is the one which has been formative of Western concepts of life, death and medical care.

I hope I have not appeared to suppose that the surgeon, or medical scientist, is always right and the public always blind to what is good for it. On the contrary, I would insist that there must always be an appeal of some sort to what I must call 'the humane consciousness' of mankind if we are to discern between the legitimate and the illegitimate in medical as in other scientific research and practice. It is this sort of appeal which has given us, in recent years, the codes of Nuremburg, Geneva and Helsinki. Ethics does not proceed from the belief that men are angels; but it does not suppose them to be devils either. And that fundamental belief in a moral consciousness in man to which an appeal can be made is perhaps the most valuable product of that very tradition which I have been talking about. To this, therefore, I make my appeal when we discuss the ethical problems facing our own, mixed society. I have tried to distinguish some elements in the Hebraic-Christian tradition which have become embedded, by historical processes, in the common stock of contemporary humanism.

REFERENCES

1. D. S. Wallace-Hadrill, *The Greek Patristic view of Nature.* (Manchester University Press, 1968, p. 67)

2. See *Decisions About Life and Death: A Problem in Modern Medicine.* C.I.O. (London, 1965)